Anshan Gold Standard Mini Atlas Series
Fetal Anomalies

System requirement:
- **Windows XP or above**
- **Power DVD player (Software)**
- **Windows Media Player version 10.0 or above**
- **Quick time player version 6.5 or above**

Accompanying CD ROM is playable only in Computer and not in CD player.

Kindly wait for few seconds for CD to autorun. If it does not autorun then please do the following:
- Click on my computer
- Click the **drive labelled JAYPEE** and after opening the drive, kindly double click the file **Jaypee**

Anshan Gold Standard Mini Atlas Series

Fetal Anomalies

Kuldeep Singh
MBBS FAUI FICMCH FICMU
Consultant Ultrasonologist
Special Interest in Obstetric Sonology
in Detailed Anomaly Scanning and
Color Doppler for Management and Gynecological Scan
Conducts FOGSI recognised ultrasound training course
Obstetrics, Gynecology and Infertility
(Basics, Color Doppler, 3D & 4D)
Dr Kuldeep's Ultrasound and Color Doppler Clinic
D 80, East of Kailash
New Delhi 110065, India
Phones: 011-26441720, 26233342
Mobile: 9811196613
singhdrkuldeep@rediffmail.com

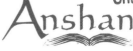

Anshan

Tunbridge Wells
UK

JAYPEE BROTHERS
MEDICAL PUBLISHERS (P) LTD.
New Delhi

First published in the UK by

Anshan Ltd
in 2008
6 Newlands Road
Tunbridge Wells
Kent TN4 9AT, UK

Tel: +44 (0)1892 557767
Fax: +44 (0)1892 530358
E-mail: info@anshan.co.uk
www.anshan.co.uk

ISBN 10   1-905740-25-5
ISBN 13   978-1-905740-25-3

British Library Cataloguing in Publication Data
A catalogue record for this book is available from the British Library

Printed in India by Ajanta Offset & Packagings Ltd., New Delhi

Many of the designations used by manufacturers and sellers to distinguish their
products are claimed as trademarks. Where those designations appear in this book
and where the publisher was aware of a trademark claim, the designations have
been printed in initial capital letters.

*This book is dedicated
to my parents*
*Mrs. Yoginder Kaur
Mr. K.J. Singh
who are with God*

*In Fond
Remembrance of
My Dear Pet Suzi*

Preface

Ultrasound in antenatal screening is an essential part of the protocol for antenatal care. It is used for fetal viability and well-being but the most important part is detection of congenital anomalies. With technological advancements and newer techniques one can use this modality for early detection of anomalies. The emotional and financial stress on the parents and society can be reduced by the judicious use of the technique.

One must still understand the limitations of the technique and that many advancements are yet to come.

This book will help everybody who is dealing with antenatal care to interpret and understand the anomalies and give their patients specific information of what to expect. Multiple pictures for all anomalies have been given for a simple and practical understanding.

It has been a sincere endeavour to make it a helpful reference book.

Kuldeep Singh

Acknowledgements

This book would never have been possible without the help of my seniors and well wishers who have stood by me and given me the confidence and the driving force to accomplish these feats. Special mention for Dr Narendra Malhotra and Dr Jaideep Malhotra (Agra), Dr PK Shah (Mumbai), Dr Bhupendra Ahuja (Agra), Dr Satpal Gupta and Dr Kamal Gupta (Jalandhar).

Special thanks to my teacher Dr Ashok Khurana and my seniors in Delhi, Dr RN Bagga, Dr Varun Duggal, and Dr Renu Caprihan.

The patience that my family has shown in bearing my absence from their time is phenomenal. Nishu K Singh my wife and my children Jaanvi Sana Chhabra and Ramanjeet Singh, thank you very much for sparing me on those late evenings and Sundays.

Contents

Chapter 1

Head and Brain
(Normal Anatomy)

CRANIAL BIOMETRY (TRANSTHALAMIC VIEW)

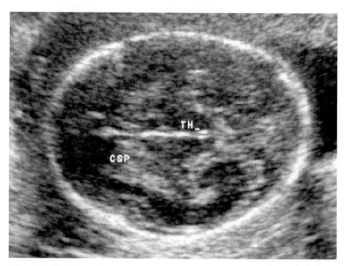

Fig. 1.1: Section for cranial biometry consisting of the thalamus, the third ventricle and the cavum septum pellucidum. The biparietal diameter is the side to side measurement from the outer table of the proximal skull to the inner table of the distal skull. The head perimeter is the the total cranial circumference, which includes the maximum anteroposterior diameter. The occipito-frontal diameter is the front to back measurement from the outer table on both sides

VENTRICULAR ATRIUM (TRANSVENTRICULAR VIEW)

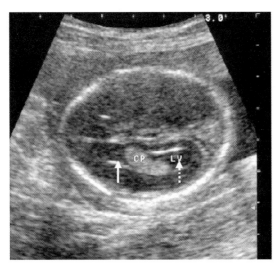

Fig. 1.2: Choroid plexus (CP) seen occupying the whole of the body of the lateral ventricle (LV). The anterior horn of the lateral ventricle (solid arrow) seen on the left side and posterior horn of the lateral ventricle (dashed arrow) seen on the right side are not filled by the choroid plexus

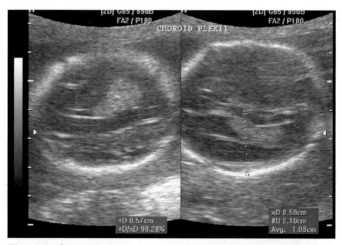

Fig. 1.3: Choroid plexus seen in the lateral ventricles on both sides

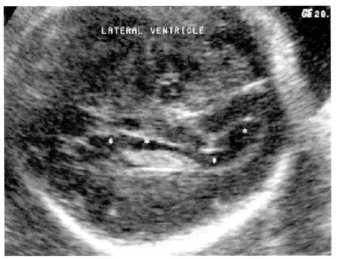

Fig. 1.4: The choroid plexus quite often does not occupy the whole of the body of the lateral ventricle and the frontal and the posterior horn also are not filled by the choroid plexus (stars)

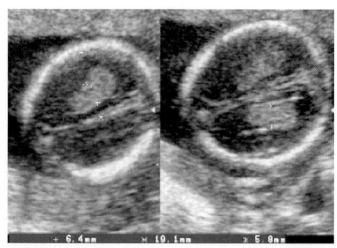

Fig. 1.5: The width of the body of the lateral ventricle, the interhemispheric distance and the ratio of the width of the body of the lateral ventricle to the interhemispheric distance is calculated (Normal value < 50%). This is not sensitive for early hydrocephalus. The width of the body, anterior horn and posterior horn of the lateral ventricle are taken (Normal value < 08 mm, borderline 08-10 mm and > 10 mm abnormal)

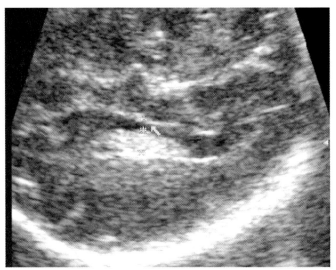

Fig. 1.6: When the choroid plexus does not occupy the whole of the body of the lateral ventricle see for the measurement of the medial separation (arrow) of the choroid plexus from the wall of the lateral ventricle (Normal value < 02 mm, borderline 02-03 mm and > 03 mm is abnormal)

CEREBELLUM (TRANSCEREBELLAR VIEW)

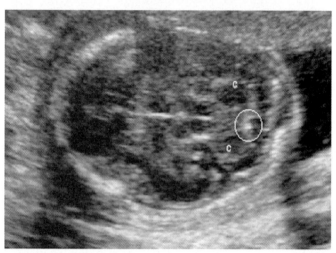

Fig. 1.7: The cerebellum is seen as a 'W' turned 90 degrees. The cerebellar hemispheres (C) and the cerebellar vermis (within the circle) should be appreciated for posterior cranial fossa abnormalities

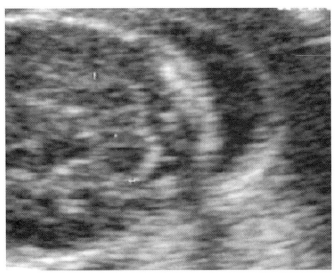

Fig. 1.8: The cerebellar transverse diameter (CTD) is measured from the edges of both cerebellar hemispheres. The CTD in mm from 14-22 weeks is equal to the gestational age of the fetus in weeks

CISTERNA MAGNA

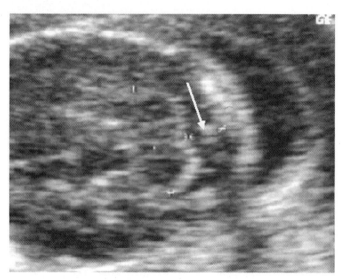

Fig. 1.9: The cisterna magna is seen posterior to the cerebellar vermis and anterior to the occipital bone (solid arrow) (Normal value < 08 mm, borderline 08-10 mm and > 10 mm abnormal). Few strands seen traversing the cisterna magna are normal. Carefully check for any communication between the fourth ventricle and the cisterna magna with an abnormal cerebellar vermis. If there is any communication at gestational age less than 16 weeks revaluate the fetus after 2 weeks

Chapter 2

Anomalies of the Head and Brain

EXENCEPHALY (ACRANIA)

• Partial or complete absence of cranial vault (Fig. 2.1).

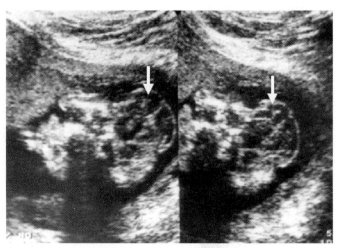

Fig. 2.1: Deformed cranium with almost no osseous area surrounding the floating brain (solid arrows)

- Brain tissue (disorganized) always present.
- Can be diagnosed on transvaginal scan at 10½ weeks (Fig. 2.2).

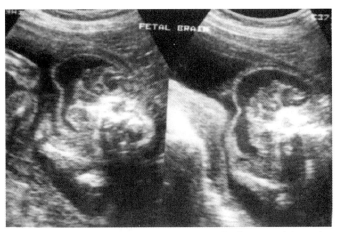

Fig. 2.2: Acrania; diagnosed on a transvaginal scan at 11 weeks. There is an absence of the cranial vault with brain tissue seen floating in the liquor

ANENCEPHALY

- The cranial vault and telencephalon are absent and the brainstem and parts of the mesencephalon are present which are covered by a vascular membrane.
- Failure to identify normal bony structure and brain tissue cephalad to the bony orbits is the most reliable feature of this anomaly (Figs 2.3 and 2.4).

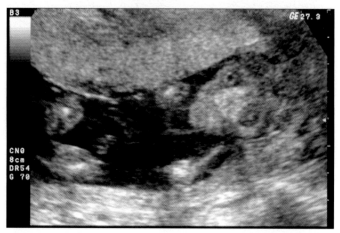

Fig. 2.3: Orbits (arrow heads) seen with nothing seen superior to it (neither brain nor bone)

- Diagnosis can be made as early as 10-11 weeks of gestation by a transvaginal scan.

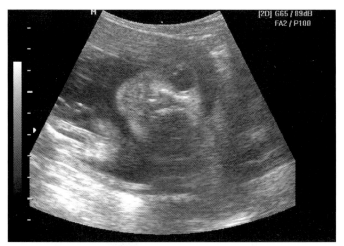

Fig. 2.4: Fetal face in an anencephalic fetus

ENCEPHALOCELE

- Mostly occurs in the midline in the occipital area.
- Can occasionally occur in the parietal and frontal bones.
- The defect in the bony skull can be demonstrated on ultrasound (Figs 2.5 and 2.6).

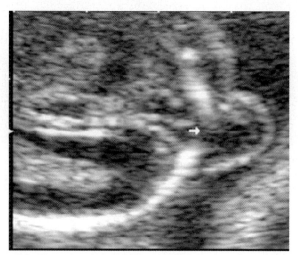

Fig. 2.5: Note the defect in the occipital bone (arrow) with the herniation of brain tissue from the defect

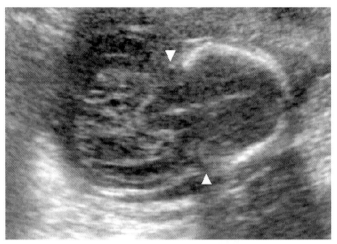

Fig. 2.6: Large defect (arrow heads) in the cranium with most of the brain tissue herniating through the defect

- Can be a meningocele, meningomyelocele, encephalo-meningocele (Fig. 2.7) or encephalocystomeningocele depending on the contents within the herniation.

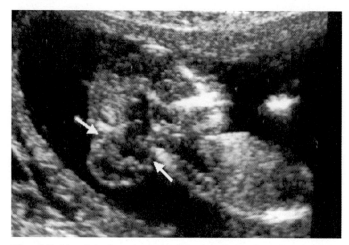

Fig. 2.7: Herniated contents (solid arrows) overhanging the fetal neck

- Assess for any hydrocephalus (Fig. 2.8).
- When the lesion is large it can cause microcephaly.
- Common associations in the cranium can be agenesis of corpus callosum, Dandy-Walker malformation.
- Renal, facial, skeletal and cardiac abnormalities can be other common associations.
- Prognosis depends on the site, size and content of lesion and associated abnormalities.

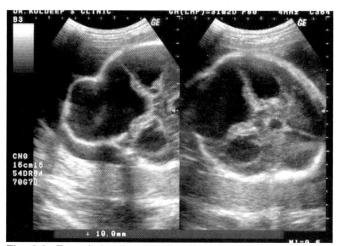

Fig. 2.8: Encephalocele with dilatation of the lateral ventricles and third ventricle

INIENCEPHALY

- There is a bony defect in the occipital region of the skull with a partial or total absence of the cervical and thoracic vertebra with spina bifida and a fixed retroflexion of the head (Figs 2.9 and 2.10).

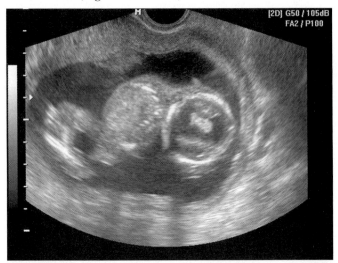

Fig. 2.9: Iniencephaly with a fixed retroflexion deformity of the fetal head

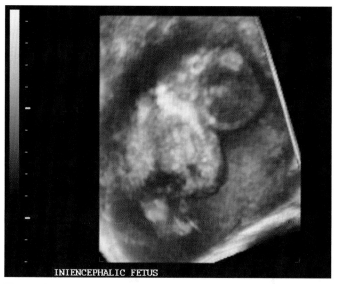

INIENCEPHALIC FETUS

Fig. 2.10: Iniencephaly as seen on 3D

ALOBAR

- Interhemispheric fissure and the falx cerebri are totally absent.
- There is a single primitive ventricle (holoventricle).
- Dorsal sac between skull and cerebral convexity can be seen (Fig. 2.11).

21

- Thalami are fused in the midline.
- Third ventricle, neurohypophysis, olfactory bulbs and tracts are absent.
- The midbrain, brainstem and cerebellum are structurally normal.
- Invariably poor prognosis.

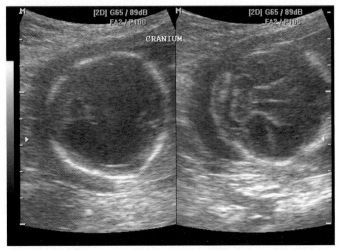

Fig. 2.11: Alobar holoprosencephaly: Dorsal sac with a mono-ventricular cavity

SEMILOBAR

- Monoventricular cavity with rudimentary occipital horns is seen.
- Falx and interhemispheric fissure form caudally with partial separation of occipital lobes.
- Thalami fused in midline (Fig. 2.12).
- Olfactory bulbs and corpus callosum usually absent.
- Dorsal sac between skull and cerebral convexity can be seen.
- Invariably poor prognosis.
- IUD or NND and those who survive have severe mental retardation.

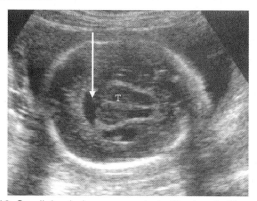

Fig. 2.12: Semilobar holoprosencephaly: Single primitive ventricle (holoventricle) (solid arrow) seen with thalami (T) fused in the midline

LOBAR

- Septum pellucidum is absent.
- Interhemispheric fissure is well-developed posteriorly (Fig. 2.13).
- The outcome depends on the severity of hydrocephalus affecting the neurologic development.
- Patients could vary from a near normal intellectual development to severe mental retardation.

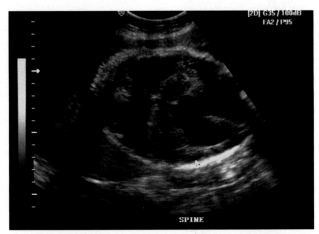

Fig. 2.13: Lobar holoprosencephaly: The septum pellucidum is absent but the inter-hemispheric fissure is well-developed posteriorly

- Cyclopia (No nose or median facial bones), proboscis, monophthalmia or anophthalmia can be seen.
- Ethmocephaly (severe hypotelorism with a proboscis), cebocephaly (hypotelorism with the nose present) are other facial deformities of various intensities that can be seen (Figs 2.14 and 2.15).

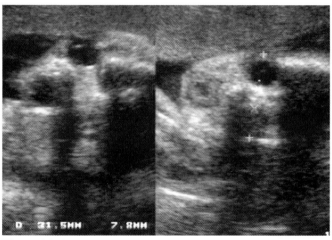

Fig. 2.14: Hypotelorism seen in a case of semilobar holo-prosencephaly. The ocular diameter in this case was 12 mm, the interocular distance was 08 mm and the binocular distance was 32 mm

- Cleft lip and palate can be seen.
- Normal cranial size, microcephaly (in alobar and semilobar varieties) or macrocephaly (because of hydrocephalus) can be seen as well.
- Polydactyly of hands and feet are common skeletal deformities.
- Other systems that can be affected are renal (dysplasia), gastrointestinal (omphalocele, esophageal atresia) and cardiac.
- Polyhydramnios and intrauterine growth retardation can be seen.
- Strong association with trisomy 13.

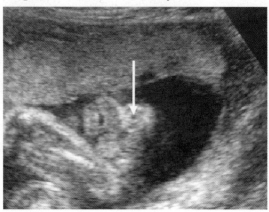

Fig. 2.15: Single nostril (solid arrow) seen in the case of hypotelorism with semilobar holoprosencephaly

COMPLETE AGENESIS OF CORPUS CALLOSUM

- The ventricles are displaced laterally with indentation of the medial walls.
- Ventriculomegaly seen in the atrial and occipital regions (colpocephaly) because of poorly developed white matter surrounding these areas (Tear drop configuration) (Fig. 2.16).

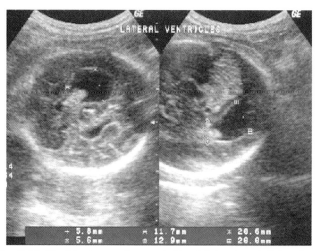

Fig. 2.16: Ventriculomegaly seen in the atrial and occipital regions (colpocephaly) because of poorly developed white matter surrounding these areas (Tear drop configuration) with an absent cavum septum pellucidum

- Enlarged elevated third ventricle between the hemispheres is seen as an inter-hemispheric cyst.
- Cavum septum pellucidum is absent.

DANDY-WALKER MALFORMATION

- Enlarged posterior fossa/deep cisterna magna is seen (Fig. 2.17).

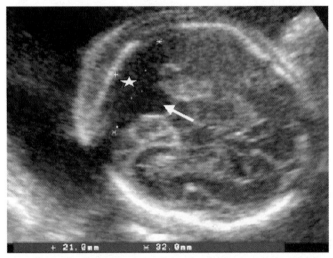

Fig. 2.17: Large cyst in the posterior cranial fossa (star) with a hypoplastic cerebellar vermis (solid arrow)

Anomalies of the Head and Brain

- Midline cyst in the posterior cranial fossa communicating with the fourth ventricle.
- Cerebellar vermis is either absent or small or abnormally developed (Fig. 2.18).
- Hydrocephalus is seen quite commonly.

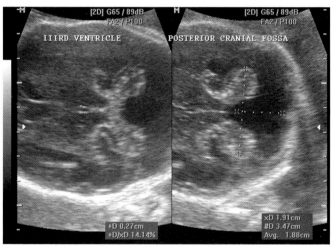

Fig. 2.18: Abnormally developed cerebellar vermis (arrow heads)

HYDRANENCEPHALY

- Can result from a bilateral *in utero* internal carotid artery occlusion or cytomegalovirus or toxoplasmosis infection.
- Complete or almost complete destruction of cerebral cortex and basal ganglia with intact meninges and skull of normal appearance (Fig. 2.19).
- They are usually stillborn or die soon after birth.

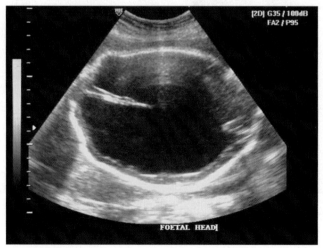

Fig. 2.19: Hydranencephaly with complete destruction of the cerebral cortex and basal ganglia with intact meninges and skull which is of normal appearance

VEIN OF GALEN ANEURYSM

- Aneurysmal dilatation of the vein of Galen is seen which lies within the subarachnoid space posterior and superior to the thalami.
- One sees a midline cyst with flow (Fig. 2.20) of an arteriovenous malformation which is diagnostic.
- Hydrocephalus can be seen.

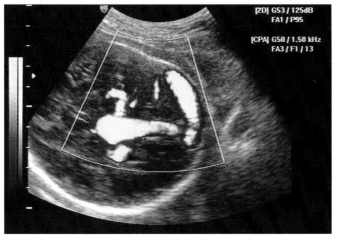

Fig. 2.20: Vein of Galen aneurysm as seen on power angio

CHOROID PLEXUS CYSTS

- Seen as thin-walled clear cysts which can be single or multiple, unilateral or bilateral (Figs 2.21 and 2.22).
- Frequently associated with trisomy 18 and sometimes with trisomy 21.

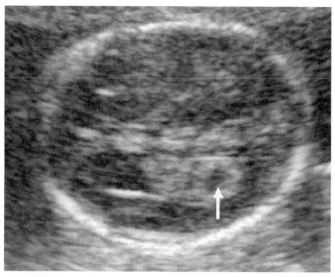

Fig. 2.21: Unilateral single (solid arrow) choroid plexus cyst

- A detailed scan to check for sonographic stigmata of chromosomal abnormalities especially trisomy 18 is done and only if any additional anomaly is detected an amniocentesis is indicated for.

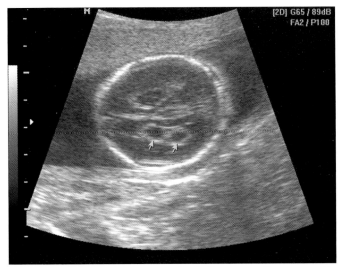

Fig. 2.22: Two choroid plexus cysts, both seen on the same side

VENTRICULOMEGALY

- Ventriculomegaly refers to an enlargement of the lateral ventricles.
- The width of the body, anterior horn and posterior horn of the lateral ventricle are taken (Normal value < 08 mm, borderline 08-10 mm and > 10 mm abnormal) (Fig. 2.23).

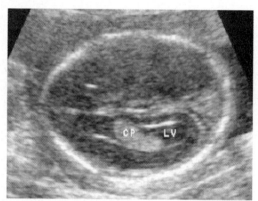

Fig. 2.23: Choroid plexus (CP) seen occupying the whole of the body of the lateral ventricle (LV). The width of the body, anterior horn and posterior horn of the lateral ventricle are taken (Normal value < 08 mm, borderline 08-10 mm and > 10 mm abnormal) When the choroid plexus does not occupy the whole of the body of the lateral ventricle see for the measurement of the medial separation of the choroid plexus from the wall of the lateral ventricle (Normal value < 02 mm, borderline 02-03 mm and > 03 mm is abnormal)

- An additional sonographic sign of ventriculomegaly is loss of approximation between the choroid plexus and the medial border of the lateral ventricle. In early stages of ventriculomegaly the choroid plexuses are seen detached from the medial wall. When the choroid plexus does not occupy the whole of the body of the

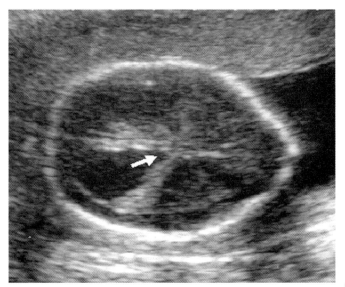

Fig. 2.24: Enlarged lateral ventricles with loss of the approximation between the choroid plexus and the medial border of the lateral ventricle (solid arrow)

35

lateral ventricle see for the measurement of the medial separation of the choroid plexus from the wall of the lateral ventricle (Normal value < 02 mm, borderline 02-03 mm and > 03 mm is abnormal) (Figs 2.24 and 2.25).

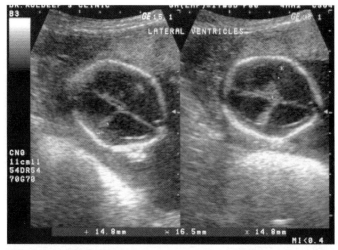

Fig. 2.25: The choroid plexuses seen detached from the medial wall in ventriculomegaly

- The cerebrospinal fluid flows through foramen of Monro to the third ventricle, and obstruction at this level results in ventriculomegaly with a normal third ventricle.
- If obstruction occurs at the level of aqueduct of Sylvius both lateral ventricles and third ventricle are dilated (Fig. 2.26).

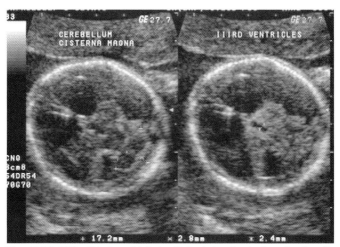

Fig. 2.26: If the third ventricle is dilated check whether the fourth ventricle is dilated or not and whether the posterior cranial fossa structures are adequately visualized or not

- A careful evaluation of the spine should always be performed once ventriculomegaly is diagnosed.
- In a communicating hydrocephalus there is overlapping of frontal bones (lemon shape) (Fig. 2.27) and downward displacement of cerebellum (banana sign) (Fig. 2.28).

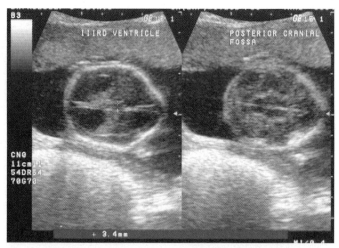

Fig. 2.27: If the posterior cranial fossa structures are not adequately visualized one should be reasonably sure that there is some sort of spinal anomaly

- Other causes of ventriculomegaly include: choroid plexus papilloma, intracranial hemorrhage, agenesis of corpus callosum, lissencephaly, Dandy-Walker malformation and congenital infections with cytomegalovirus or toxoplasmosis.
- The prognosis depends upon the underlying cause of ventriculomegaly and the type and severity of associated malformations.

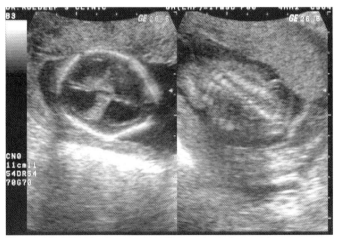

Fig. 2.28: Ventriculomegaly with a spinal dysraphism

Chapter 3

Fetal Face
(Normal Anatomy)

BASICS

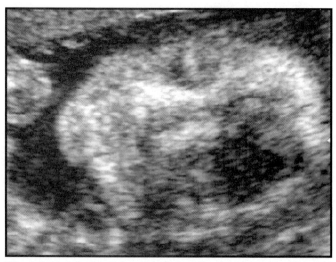

Fig. 3.1: Detailed facial anatomy which can be seen in a second trimester ultrasound. Note the eyelids, nose, lips, cheeks and chin which can be seen so clearly and can be shown to the expectant parents as well

ORBITS AND LENS

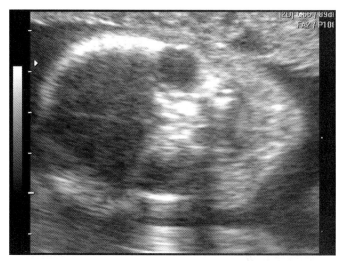

Fig. 3.2: View for the measurements of ocular diameter (measured from medial inner to medial lateral wall of the orbit), interocular distance (measured from medial inner wall of one orbit to medial inner wall of the other orbit) and binocular distance (measured from lateral inner wall of one orbit to lateral inner wall of the other orbit)

43

LIPS, MAXILLA, MANDIBLE, NASAL BONE AND TONGUE

- Modified coronal view for the lips and maxilla.
- 3D ultrasound is more beneficial for evaluating facial malformations (Figs 3.3 and 3.4).
- Surface display rendering and multiplanar reconstruction in three planes defines facial malformations much better.

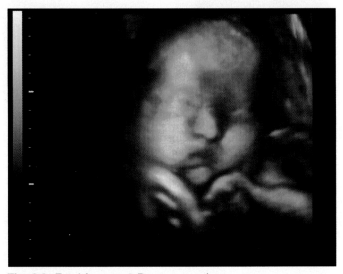

44 **Fig. 3.3:** Fetal face on 3 D reconstruction

- Axial plane view for the maxilla and soft tissue overlying it and the tooth-bearing alveolar ridge.

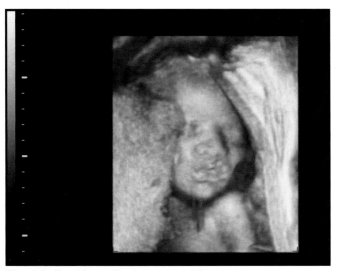

Fig. 3.4: Fetal face clearly seen on 3D

- For nasal bone mid-sagittal view of the fetal profile should be obtained (Fig. 3.5).
- Nasal bone echogenecity should be greater than overlying skin.

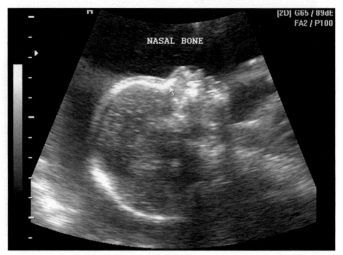

Fig. 3.5: Nasal bone echogenecity should be greater than overlying skin. Correct view of the nasal bone demonstrates three lines. Two parallel lines which are proximal to the forehead (equal sign). The third line at a higher level represents the tip of the nose

- Longitudinal (facial profile) view and transverse view of the mandible, tongue, hard palate and nasal bridge (Fig 3.6).

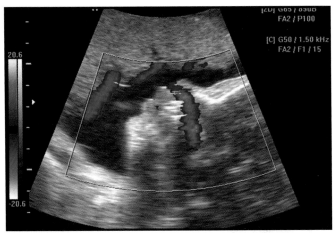

Fig. 3.6: Normal palate seen with color flow imaging with respiratory activity showing movement in the nasopharynx superior to an intact palate

Ears

- Usually the ear in the near field if outlined by amniotic fluid is usually visible.
- Fetal ear in the far field especially if the fetus lies in the lateral position is difficult to visualize.
- Rescan after few minutes for change of fetal position and try and delineate the ear by a coronal approach of the cranium.
- Coronal and parasagittal (modified longitudinal plane) views are taken (Fig. 3.7).

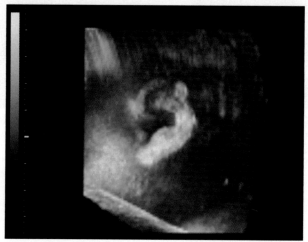

48 **Fig. 3.7:** Fetal ear as shown on 3D reconstruction

Chapter 4

Fetal Facial Anomalies

CLEFT AND PALATE

- The cleft can be incomplete/complete, unilateral/
  bilateral, lateral/midline and symmetric/asymmetric
  (Figs 4.1 to 4.4).
- Clefts can involve
  1. Only the upper lip.
  2. Upper lip and the anterior portion of the maxilla.
  3. Upper lip, the anterior portion of the maxilla and
     the posterior portion of the palate.
  4. Only the posterior portion of the palate.

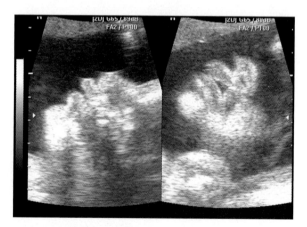

Fig. 4.1: Unilateral cleft lip

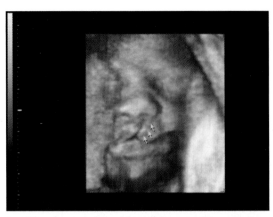

Fig. 4.2: 3D reconstruction of the cleft upper lip as shown on 2D in Figure 4.1. This helps the parents to understand better

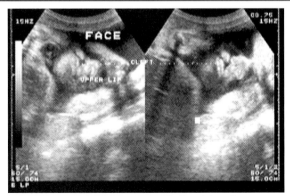

Fig. 4.3: Unilateral cleft in the upper lip involving the nose as well

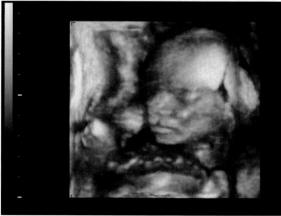

Fig. 4.4: 3D reconstruction of the bilateral cleft lip as seen from the side

- The bilateral cleft lip and palate variety are the easiest to be diagnosed as they are easily recognizable sonographically on all routine 2D views for the face (Figs 4.5 and 4.6).

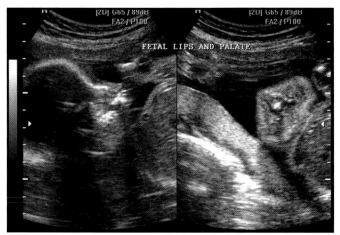

Fig. 4.5: Bilateral cleft lip as seen on the profile view to show upward extension and end on view to show inner extension

- Unilateral cleft lip and palate can be diagnosed by a coronal and sagittal view.
- Median cleft lip is also seen by the modified coronal view.

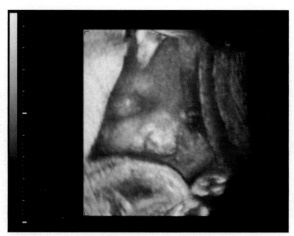

Fig. 4.6: Bilateral cleft lip as seen on 3D reconstruction

HYPOTELORISM (FIGS 4.7 AND 4.8)

- The interocular distance and binocular distance are below 2 standard deviations of the mean (Fig. 4.7).
- Most commonly associated with holoprosencephaly (Fig. 4.8).
- Associated facial abnormalities like cebocephaly and cleft lip and palate should also be looked for.

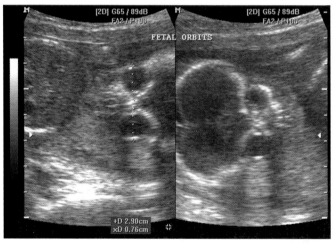

Fig. 4.7: Hypotelorism seen in a case of semilobar holoprosencephaly. The ocular diameter in this case was 12 mm, the interocular distance was 08 mm and the binocular distance was 29 mm

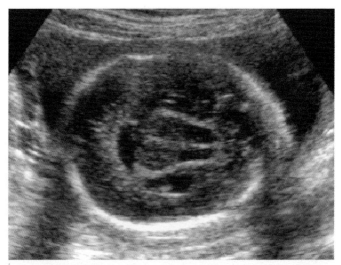

Fig. 4.8: Semilobar holoprosencephaly with associated hypotelorism

MICROGNATHIA

- Seen as a small mandible with a receding chin (Fig. 4.9)

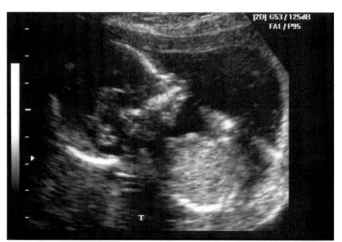

Fig. 4.9: Micrognathia (receding chin) seen in a case of trisomy 18

- Midline sagittal view or profile view (Fig. 4.10) is the most helpful to evaluate the size of mandible in respect to the face.

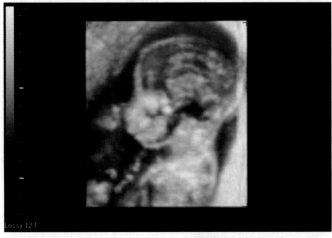

Fig. 4.10: Fetal mandible as seen normally on a sagittal scan

MICROPHTHALMIA

- It is seen as a small globe which is confirmed by orbital measurements.
- Can be detected in the early second trimester when orbital measurements are taken (Fig. 4.11).

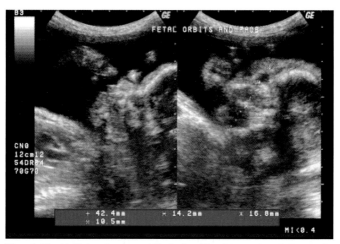

Fig. 4.11: Unilateral microphthalmia. The binocular distance is 42.4 mm, the interocular distance is 16 mm, the left ocular diameter is 14 mm and the right ocular diameter is 10 mm

NASAL BONE

- Visualized in the mid-sagittal view in fetal profile with adequate magnification.
- In continuation with nuchal translucency, ductus venosus and biochemical markers absence of nasal bone indicates possibility of a chromosomal abnormality most common being trisomy 21 (Figs 4.12 and 4.13).

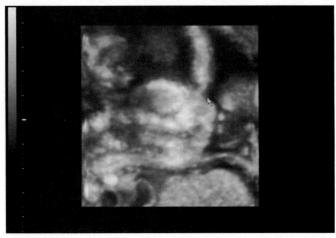

Fig. 4.12: Absent nasal bone (arrow)

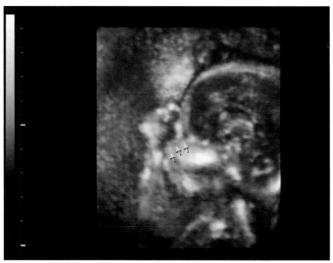

Fig. 4.13: Absent nasal bone as seen in the profile view. This can be associated with various aneuploidies especially trisomy 21

Chapter 5

Fetal Neck
(Normal Anatomy)

NUCHAL TRANSLUCENCY

- Posteriorly nuchal translucency (Fig. 5.1) or nuchal skin fold thickness is assessed through the section for the cerebellum and cisterna magna (Fig. 5.2) or just inferior to it for skin and soft tissues overlying the neck (Fig. 5.3).

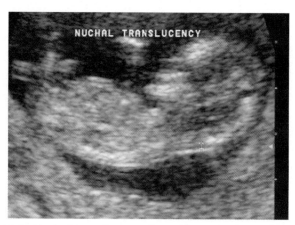

Fig. 5.1: Nuchal translucency in a 13 weeks fetus. Nuchal translucency thickness usually increases with gestational age with 1.5 mm and 2.5 mm being the 50th and 95th percentile respectively for gestational ages between 10 and 12 weeks. 2.0 mm and 3.0 mm are the 50th and 95th percentile respectively for gestational ages between 12 and 14 weeks

NUCHAL SKIN FOLD

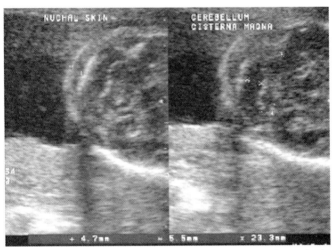

Fig. 5.2: Nuchal skin fold thickness assessment through the section for the cerebellum and cisterna magna

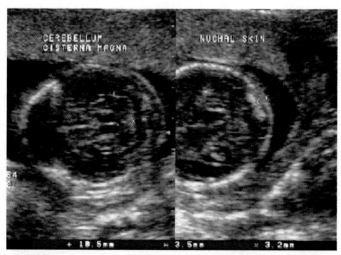

Fig. 5.3: Nuchal skin fold thickness assessment through the section just inferior to the section for cerebellum and cisterna magna (14-18 weeks : Normal value < 04 mm, Borderline 04-05 mm and > 05 mm requires further karyotypic analysis) (18-22 weeks : Normal value < 05 mm, Borderline 05-06 mm and > 06 mm requires further karyotypic analysis)

Chapter 6

Anomalies of the Fetal Neck

CYSTIC HYGROMA

- It is collection of fluid in the soft tissue of the neck caused due to local lymphedema.
- Can be seen characteristically in the longitudinal section of the spine at the craniovertebral junction and cervical area (Figs 6.1 and 6.2).
- They are seen as a localized lesion in the cervical area or can be seen as a diffuse lesion on the thorax and abdomen.

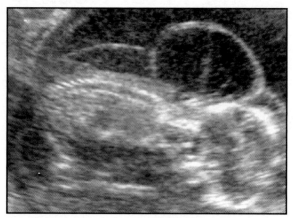

Fig. 6.1: Cystic hygroma seen in the longitudinal section across the entire fetal spine

- Cysts can be small/large or septated/nonseptated.
- Can be diagnosed in late first trimester and early second trimester.

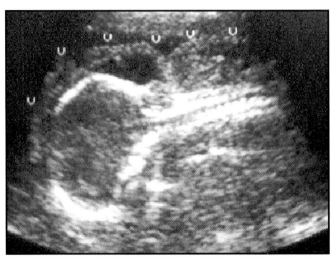

Fig. 6.2: Cystic hygroma seen in the longitudinal section posterior to the cranium, craniovertebral junction and cervical vertebra

Chapter 7

Fetal Spine
(Normal Anatomy)

BASICS

- At 16 weeks of gestation the vertebrae can be delineated individually on ultrasound by looking at the ossification centers in the transverse plane. These are echogenic and are three in number with two of them posterior and one anterior (Fig. 7.1).
- The cutaneous, subcutaneous and muscular components seen posterior to the vertebral column need to be carefully screened all along the cervical, dorsal, lumbar, sacral and coccygeal spine.

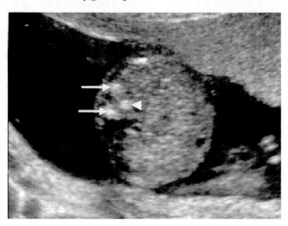

Fig. 7.1: Three ossification centers seen in the transverse plane. Two of these are posterior (solid arrows) and one is anterior (arrow head)

- All three planes the longitudinal, sagittal and transverse planes need to be viewed in every case through all the vertebrae.

LONGITUDINAL PLANES

- The longitudinal and transverse planes delineate the soft tissue components posterior to the spine and dysraphic disorganization of the spine (Fig. 7.2).

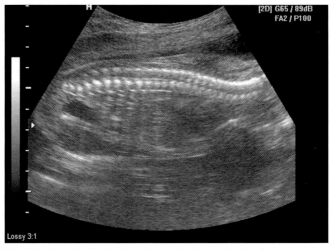

Fig. 7.2: Longitudinal plane through the entire fetal spine

SAGITTAL PLANES

- The sagittal plane delineates the spinal cord (Fig. 7.3) which is hyperechoic for any tethering or splitting or improper termination and also the vertebral column for any cartilagenous or osseous spurs (Fig. 7.4).

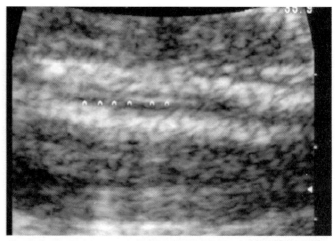

Fig. 7.3: Sagittal plane to delineate the spinal cord

- The transverse plane delineates any minimal widening of the interpedicular distance and the status of the spinal cord to the adjacent membranes.

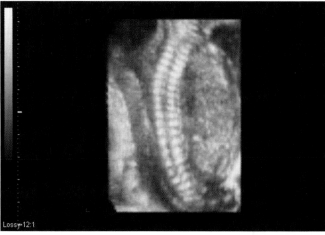

Fig. 7.4: 3D reconstruction of the fetal vertebral column

Chapter 8

Anomalies of
the Fetal Spine

SPINA BIFIDA

- This defect involves the vertebral column and spinal cord with disruption of the cutaneous and subcutaneous elements as well (Fig. 8.1).

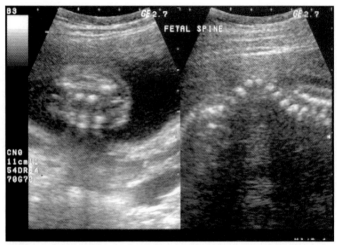

Fig. 8.1: Defect in the osseous component of the vertebral column and disruption of cutaneous and subcutaneous elements

- The osseous defect is seen as a disruption of the normal triangular appearance of the ossification centers. It can appear as a widening of the interpedicular distance (Fig. 8.2), splaying of the posterior ossification centers or a gross dysraphic disorganization.
- The affected vertebra can show a variation in the contour in comparison with one superior or inferior to it or a U-shaped configuration on transverse scanning.

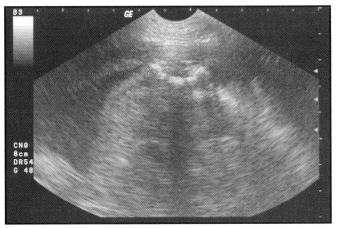

Fig. 8.2: Widening of the inter-pedicular distance

- The contents can be anechoic (meningoceles) (Fig. 8.3) or show strands or inhomogeneous tissue (meningomyelocele/lipocele).
- These defects are most commonly seen in the lumbar and lumbosacral area but can also be seen at the craniovertebral junction or the dorsal region as well.

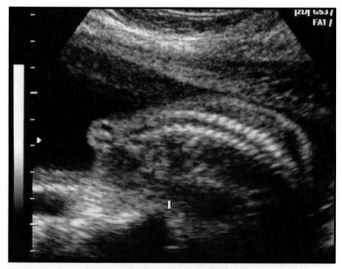

Fig. 8.3: Sacral meningocele with anechoic contents

- Carefully assess the extent of cranial involvement by checking the severity of dilatation of lateral ventricles (Fig. 8.4) and the third ventricle.
- Carefully check the delineation of posterior cranial fossa structures and the extent of herniation.
- As the cranial signs are much more evident on a routine scan do not stop at mentioning hydrocephalus. If there is dilatation of lateral ventricle and third ventricle with inadequate delineation of posterior cranial fossa structures a search for a spinal anomaly is a must.

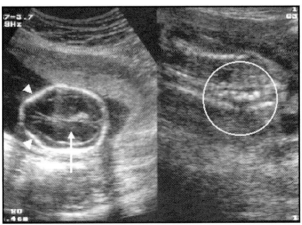

Fig. 8.4: Lumbosacral meningomyelocele (within circle) with associated dilatation of the lateral ventricles (solid arrow) and frontal bossing (lemon sign) (arrow heads)

SACROCOCCYGEAL TERATOMA

- It appears as a mass inferior to the sacrococcygeal area.
- The mass usually shows a mixed echopattern (Fig. 8.5) but can also appear as a solid mass and can be rarely cystic as well (Fig. 8.6).

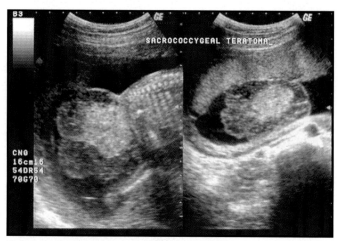

Fig. 8.5: Post-sacral mass with a mixed echopattern

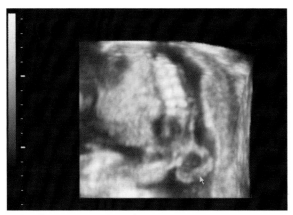

Fig. 8.6: 3D reconstruction of the post-sacral mass

- Solid areas are composed of dense tissues like cartilage and liver and also tooth and bone.
- Cystic areas are composed of soft tissues of various systems like neural, respiratory and gastrointestinal.

SCOLIOSIS AND HEMIVERTEBRA

- Lateral curvature of the spine (Fig. 8.7).
- Usually suspected when on a longitudinal section the entire spine is not properly appreciated.
- On a sagittal section the abnormal curvature is easily appreciated.
- Usually a part of spina bifida.
- Most commonly associated with a hemivertebra which is suspected as a lateral deviation of the anterior ossification center when compared with the adjacent ones.

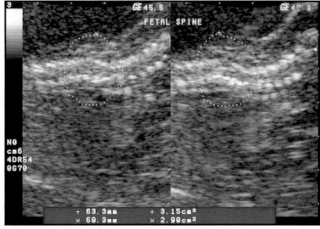

Fig. 8.7: Scoliosis (within circles) in the fetal spine

DIASTEMATOMYELIA

- Extra-echogenic posterior focus in the spinal canal (Figs 8.8 and 8.9).
- Can be seen in coronal or transverse section.

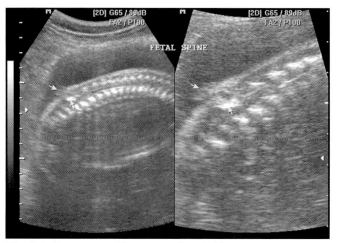

Fig. 8.8: Bony spur with an associated skin tag

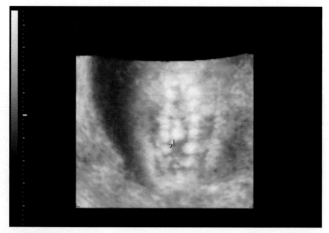

Fig. 8.9: Bony spur as seen on 3D

Chapter **9**

Fetal Thorax—
Extracardiac
(Normal Anatomy)

STRUCTURES IN THE FETAL THORAX

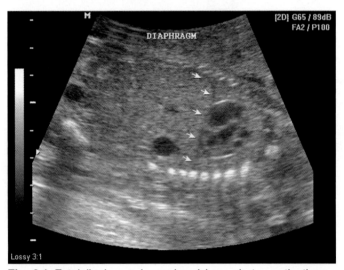

Fig. 9.1: Fetal diaphragm (arrow heads) seen between the thorax and abdomen

Table 9.1: Fetal thorax

- Diaphragm
  - Contour
  - Continuity
  - Movements
- Ribs
  - Echogenicity
  - Configuration
- Lungs
  - Echopattern
  - Lung length
- Pleura
  - Effusion
- Trachea
- Esophagus
- Masses
- Cardiothoracic ratio
- Mediastinal vasculature

Diaphragm

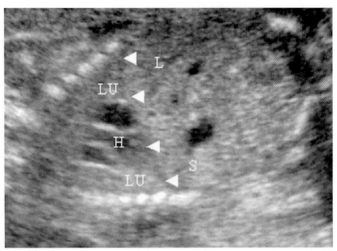

Fig. 9.2: Fetal diaphragm (arrow heads) is seen as a hypoechoic line. Superior to the diaphragm the lungs (LU) and heart (H) are seen and inferior to it the liver (L) on the right and spleen (S) on the left side are seen

Lungs

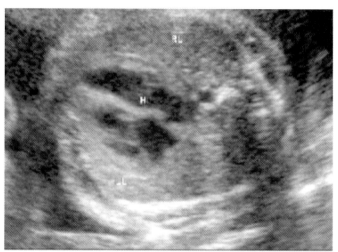

Fig. 9.3: Both fetal lungs seen in a transverse section with the heart in the center

Chapter 10

Fetal Thoracic Anomalies (Extracardiac)

PLEURAL EFFUSION

- They can be seen as anechoic fluid collections in the fetal thorax taking on the chest wall shape, diaphragmatic contour and mediastinal contour (Fig. 10.1).
- Can be unilateral or bilateral.
- Depending on the size of the effusion there may be a mediastinal displacement.
- If the effusion is large it can deform the diaphragmatic contour as well.
- Unilateral and small effusions sometimes can resolve spontaneously.

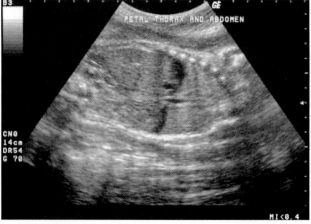

Fig. 10.1: Bilateral pleural effusion

CYSTIC ADENOMATOID MALFORMATION (FIG. 10.2)

- Can appear as a multicystic mass with cysts varying in sizes from 09 to 57 mm.
- If the cysts are extremely small it can appear as a solid mass because of distal acoustic enhancement.
- They are usually unilateral, rarely bilateral.
- Even in unilateral cases it can sometimes only affect part of the lung.
- To differentiate it from pulmonary sequestration check whether its supply is from the pulmonary artery as a sequestration has its blood supply from the systemic circulation.

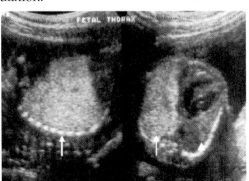

Fig. 10.2: Cystic adenomatoid malformation of the right lung (solid line). Because of distal acoustic enhancement from very small cysts the lesion appears as a solid mass. Note the difference in echo pattern from the left lung (arrow head)

LUNG SEQUESTRATION

- Can appear as a diffusely homogeneous hyperechoic mass or as an inhomogeneously hyperechoic mass with a few cystic spaces.
- Lobar or triangular in shape at the base of left fetal chest (Fig. 10.3).
- To differentiate it from a cystic adenomatoid malformation check whether its supply is from the systemic circulation (from the descending aorta and not the pulmonary artery as in cystic adenomatoid malformation).

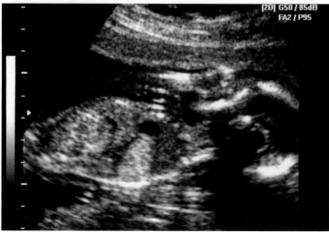

Fig. 10.3: Note the triangular shape of the sequestration at the base

CONGENITAL DIAPHRAGMATIC HERNIA

- Much more common on the left side.
- The striking feature is absent fetal stomach in the abdomen.
- A retrocardiac intrathoracic cystic mass can be seen (Figs 10.4 and 10.5).
- With bigger hernias an intestinal peristalsis can be seen.
- If the defect is even larger the spleen, left kidney and part of the liver can also be herniated in the thorax.

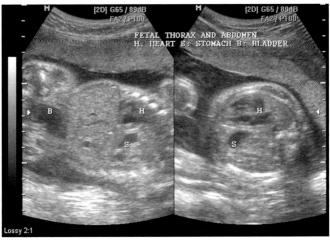

Fig. 10.4: Fetal stomach (S) seen in the retrocardiac area with the diaphragm seen

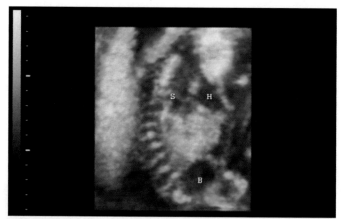

Fig. 10.5: Congenital diaphragmatic hernia as seen on 3D

- Right sided diaphragmatic hernias are much less common and involve the herniation of the liver and even less commonly bowel and the right kidney.
- It is difficult to diagnose right sided hernias because of a solid echopattern of both lung and liver.
- The diagnosis is clinched with the compression of the heart to the left side owing to a mass on the right side of the chest.
- Check the vascularity of this mass and see the vasculature (venous) superior to and inferior to the diaphragm and draining into the inferior vena cava inferiorly.

- In right sided diaphragmatic hernias the stomach is seen inferior to the diaphragm.

CONGENITAL HIGH AIRWAY OBSTRUCTION/ LARYNGEAL ATRESIA/TRACHEAL ATRESIA

- The lungs are symmetrically enlarged, echogenic, and homogeneous (Fig. 10.6).

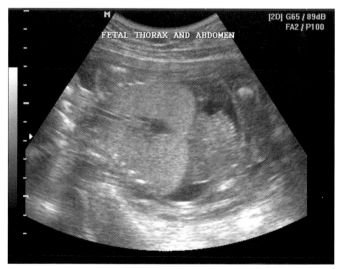

Fig. 10.6: Enlarged fetal lungs

- The distended lungs have mass effect on the diaphragm, which appears flattened or inverted, and the heart is displaced anteriorly in the midline.
- The heart often appears dwarfed by a surrounding enlarged lungs.
- Fetal ascites is almost always present at the time of diagnosis.
- Poly and oligohydramnios are reported.

Chapter 11

Fetal Heart
(Normal Anatomy)

NORMAL HEART

Fetal Heart

- Situs
- Axis
- Size
- Rate
- Rhythm
- Configuration
- Connections
- Tumors.

CARDIAC FOUR CHAMBER VIEW

- Comparative sizes of all the chambers
- Normal atrioventricular connections
- Atrioventricular malformations
- Ventricular septal defects.

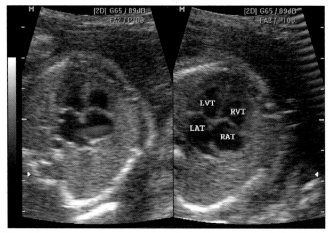

Fig. 11.1: Cardiac four chamber view. Please note that with the spine lateral or posterior one can get a good four chamber view of the heart

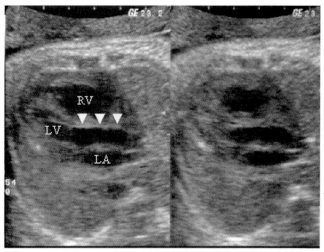

Fig. 11.2: Aorto-septal continuity (arrow heads) seen in the long axis view. The left ventricle (LV), right ventricle (RV) and left atrium (LA) are also labeled

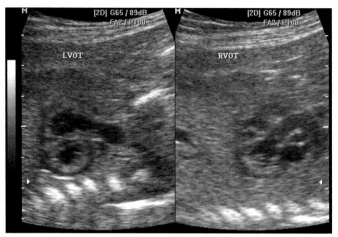

Fig. 11.3: Ventricular outflow tracts, right and left

SHORT AXIS VIEW

- Visualizes the cardiac apex through the level of the left ventricle till the mitral valve and up to the level of the great arteries.
- Right ventricular outflow tract, the pulmonary trunk with its bifurcation arising through the anterior ventricle.
- Ductus arteriosus can be seen.

Chapter 12

Anomalies of the Fetal Heart

CARDIAC ABNORMALITIES

Cardiac four chamber view
- Situs (Fig. 12.1)
- Axis

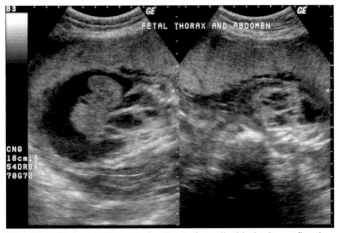

Fig. 12.1: Defect in the anterior thoracic wall with the heart floating

- Size
  - Cardiothoracic ratio (Fig. 12.2)
  - M mode ultrasound

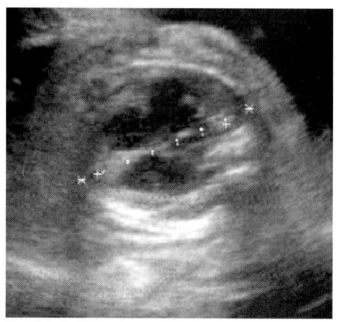

Fig. 12.2: Cardiomegaly with the cardiothoracic ratio in this case as 80 percent

- Size of ventricular chambers
  - i. Hypoplastic left ventricle or left heart (Fig. 12.3)
  - ii. Hypoplastic right ventricle

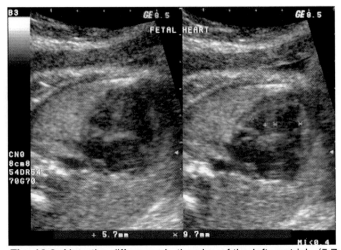

Fig. 12.3: Note the difference in the size of the left ventricle (5.7 mm) as compared to the right ventricle (9.7 mm)

- Septal defects (Fig. 12.4)
  - i. Atrial septal defect
  - ii. Ventricular septal defect
  - iii. Atrioventricular canal

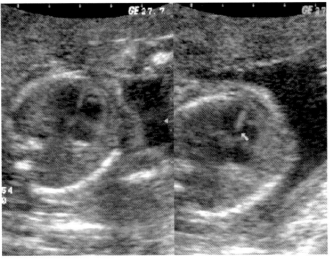

Fig. 12.4: Ventricular septal defect

- Valvular abnormalities (Fig. 12.5)
    i. Bicuspid, tricuspid, pulmonary and aortic stenosis
    ii. Bicuspid, tricuspid, pulmonary and aortic regurgitation.

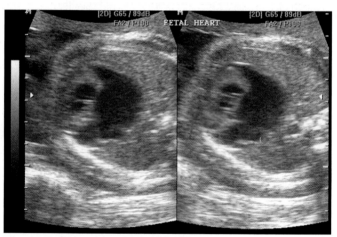

Fig. 12.5: Giant right atrium seen

- Cardiac musculature
  i. Focal thickening (Fig. 12.6)
  ii. Diffuse thickening
  iii. Change in echopattern

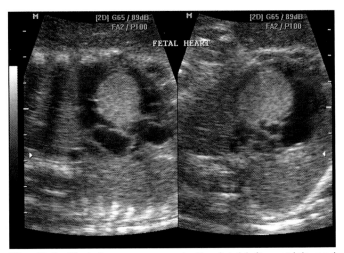

Fig. 12.6: Rhabdomyoma seen in the fetal left ventricle and obstructing the aorta partially

- Pericardial effusion (Fig. 12.7).

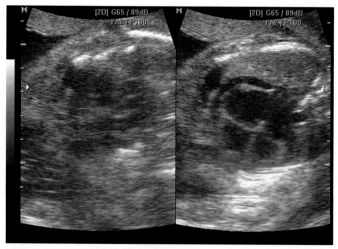

Fig. 12.7: Pericardial effusion

Chapter 13

Gastrointestinal System (Normal Anatomy)

FETAL ABDOMEN (APPROACH)

- Stomach
  - Present/Absent
  - Masses
- Duodenum
  - Double bubble
- Small bowel
  - Caliber
  - Peristalsis
- Large bowel
  - Caliber
  - Peristalsis
- Omentum/Mesentery
  - Calcification
  - Cyst
- Liver
  - Size
  - Calcification
  - Cyst
- Spleen
  - Size
  - Calcification
  - Cyst

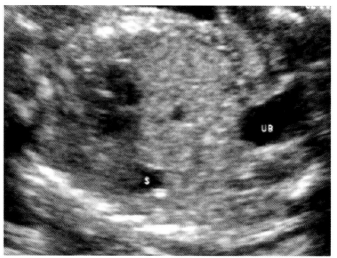

Fig. 13.1: Fluid filled structures, stomach (S) and urinary bladder (UB) seen in the fetal abdomen

PORTAL VEIN

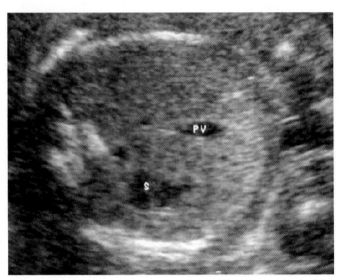

Fig. 13.2: Fluid filled structures, stomach (S) and portal vein (PV) seen in the fetal abdomen. The portal vein is usually seen in the midline and the gallbladder more on the right side

COLON

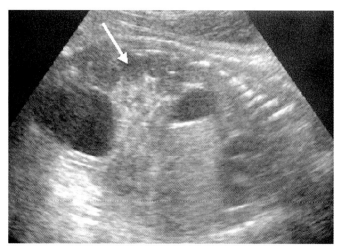

Fig. 13.3: Normal colonic echoes (hypoechoic) seen at the periphery of the fetal abdomen (solid arrow)

CYST IN FETAL ABDOMEN

- Double bubble in duodenal atresia
- Multiple fluid filled areas in jejunal and ileal atresia
- Dilated colonic loops in obstruction
- Omentum or mesentery (omental or mesenteric cyst)
- Liver (hepatic cyst)
- Biliary tree (choledochal cyst)
- Urinary bladder (obstructed)
- Kidneys (multicystic or hydronephrosis)
- Ureter (hydroureter)
- Uterus (hydrometrocolpos)
- Ovaries (cyst or teratoma)
- Spine (anterior meningocele or sacrococcygeal teratoma)
- Cloacal cyst.

Chapter 14

Anomalies of the Gastrointestinal System

ESOPHAGEAL ATRESIA

- The normal fetal esophagus can be occasionally seen on ultrasound as a tubular echogenic structure in the neck and posterior chest.
- Esophageal atresia is diagnosed by demonstration of polyhydramnios with an inability to visualize the stomach bubble (Fig. 14.1).

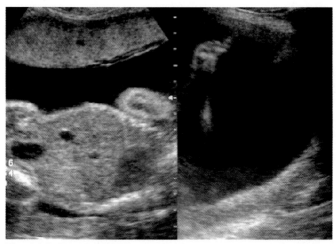

Fig. 14.1: Esophageal atresia as diagnosed by demonstration of polyhydramnios (right side) with an inability to visualize the stomach bubble (left side)

- Suspect esophageal atresia if you see polyhydramnios with IUGR.
- Proximal esophageal punch can be seen by visualizing the proximal esophageal segment.
- Without polyhydramnios if you do not see a stomach bubble rescan the patient after 30-60 minutes, if still not visible rescan the next day before you establish a diagnosis of esophageal atresia as stomach filling and emptying follows a cycle which is physiological.
- One of the most common causes of stomach bubble not seen is oligohydramnios.
- Absent stomach bubble can also be seen in diaphragmatic hernia, cleft lip and palate and CNS disorders.
- Fetuses with esophageal atresia also have a tracheoesophageal fistula and the stomach bubble can be seen if fluid crosses from the trachea into the stomach through the fistula.

DUODENAL ATRESIA

- Diagnosis of duodenal atresia is based on demonstration of a fluid-filled "double bubble" in the upper part of the fetal abdomen (Fig. 14.2).
- This is produced by a distended stomach and an enlarged duodenal bulb.

123

- Polyhydramnios is always associated with duodenal atresia.
- The double bubble sign as such is not only specific for duodenal atresia but any duodenal obstruction.

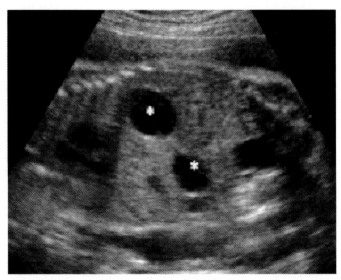

Fig. 14.2: Duodenal atresia (stars) with polyhydramnios in a case of trisomy 21

SMALL BOWEL OBSTRUCTION

- Small bowel segments usually are less than 07 mm in diameter.
- Small bowel obstruction is diagnosed by seeing multiple interconnecting, overdistended bowel loops (Fig. 14.3).
- Depending on the level of obstruction the lower the site more the number of dilated loops seen.
- Polyhydramnios is usually seen in higher level of obstruction as in jejunal and proximal ileal obstruction.

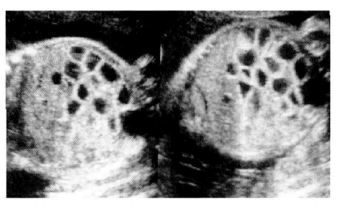

Fig. 14.3: Small bowel obstruction seen as multiple inter-connecting, overdistended bowel loops more than 07 mm in diameter. Take care that you do not confuse the same picture with a multicystic dysplastic kidney or a dilated tortuous ureter

ECHOGENIC BOWEL

- Areas of increased echogenicity in the fetal abdomen usually represent hyperechoic colonic meconium in a normal fetus at term or hyperechoic bowel contents in the fetus who has swallowed intra-amniotic blood (Fig. 14.4).

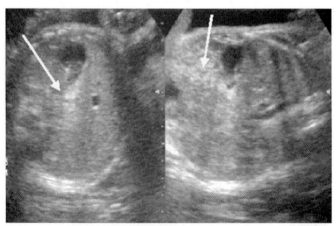

Fig. 14.4: Echogenic bowel (solid arrows) which can be normally seen in a normal fetus at term with hyperechoic colonic meconium or hyperechoic bowel contents in the fetus who has swallowed intra-amniotic blood

LARGE BOWEL OBSTRUCTION

- Large bowel obstruction is quite difficult to diagnose than small bowel obstruction.
- The biggest problem in diagnosing is lack of and variation in cut off points for diagnosing a dilated large bowel segment.
- A large bowel segment which is more than 20 mm wide near term can be termed as abnormal but the final diagnosis is made in the postnatal period (Fig. 14.5).

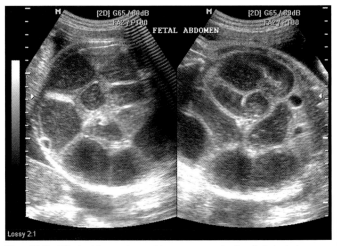

Fig. 14.5: Dilated large bowel loops seen in the fetal abdomen

GASTROSCHISIS

- It is a right paraumbilical defect involving all layers of the abdominal wall.
- Small bowel usually always herniates through the defect and multiple loops of bowel can be seen floating freely in the amniotic fluid (Fig. 14.6).
- The umbilical cord is normally inserted to the left of the defect.

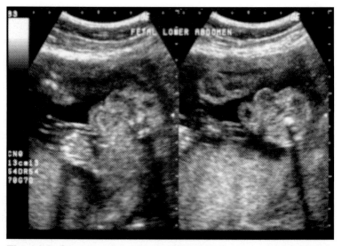

Fig. 14.6: Gastroschisis with bowel segments seen floating freely in the amniotic fluid

- Large bowel, stomach, genitourinary system and the liver can also sometimes herniate though rarely.
- Polyhydramnios can be seen sometimes.

OMPHALOCELE

- The umbilical cord enters the omphalocele.
- It is a defect of the anterior abdominal wall with extrusion of the abdominal contents into the base of the umbilical cord (Fig. 14.7).

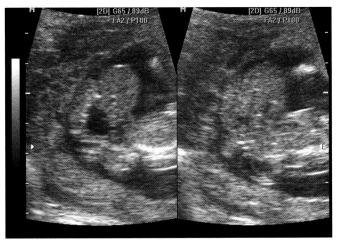

Fig. 14.7: Large omphalocele with abdominal viscera seen herniating

- An anterior midline mass containing the herniated viscera (bowel, stomach, liver) can be seen in the anterior abdominal wall defect.
- Ascites can commonly be seen.
- The size of the defect depends on the extent and type of visceral herniation into the amniotic sac.

Chapter **15**

Genitourinary Tract
(Normal Anatomy)

KIDNEYS

- Fetal kidneys develop within the pelvis at around 7 weeks of gestation.
- From 7-11 weeks the kidneys ascend to their position in the flanks.
- The kidneys excrete urine at around 11 weeks of gestation and it increases progressively which is the major contributor to the amniotic fluid volume.
- By transvaginal ultrasound fetal kidneys can be first seen as early as 9 weeks.

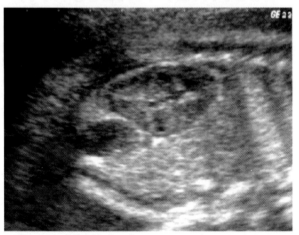

Fig. 15.1: Longitudinal scan of a normal kidney with its characteristic reniform shape

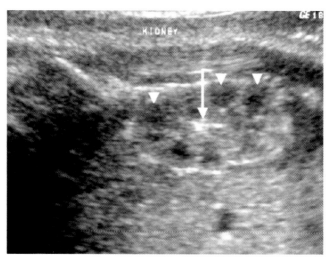

Fig. 15.2: Longitudinal scan of a normal kidney in the third trimester in a fetus of 33 weeks and 4 days. Note the central echogenic area (solid arrow) with hypoechoic pyramids (arrow heads)

- By transabdominal scanning the kidneys can be first seen at 12 to 14 weeks.
- Fetal kidneys have their characteristic reniform shape and can be seen on either side of the fetal spine and have a central echogenic area with hypoechoic pyramids (Figs 15.1 and 15.2).

- Iliacs (Fig. 17.8)

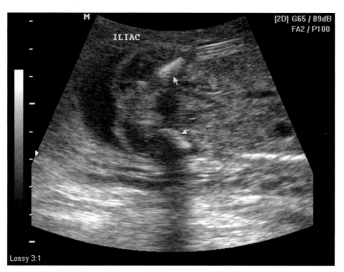

Fig. 17.8: Both iliacs to be checked for any skeletal deformities and the angle between the iliacs can be a soft marker for trisomy 21

- Femora (Fig. 17.9)

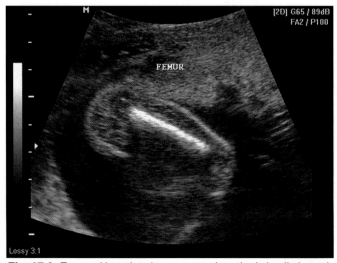

Fig. 17.9: Femoral length to be measured routinely in all obstetric ultrasound after 14 weeks

- Tibiae (Fig. 17.10)
- Fibulae (Fig. 17.10)

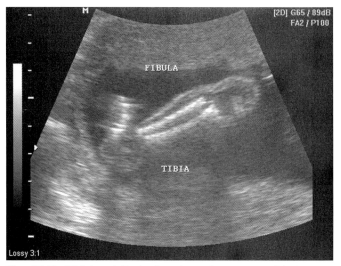

Fig. 17.10: Tibial and fibular lengths to be measured in fetuses where a skeletal deformity is being suspected

- Feet (Fig. 17.11)

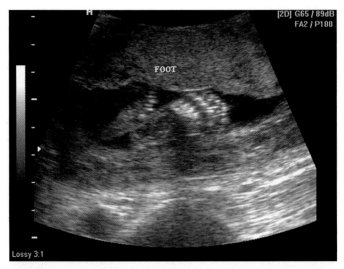

Fig. 17.11: Fetal feet to be checked for their orientation with the tibia to make a diagnosis of clubfoot

- Humerii (Fig. 17.12)

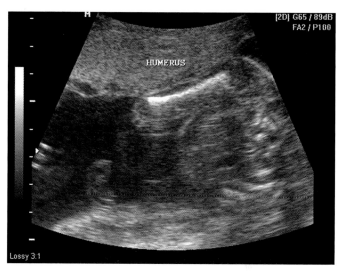

Fig. 17.12: Humeral length to be measured in all anomaly targeted obstetric ultrasound especially for chromosomal abnormalities after 14 weeks. If a skeletal deformity is being suspected the radial and ulnar lengths also to be taken

- Radii (Fig. 17.13)
- Ulnae (Fig. 17.13)

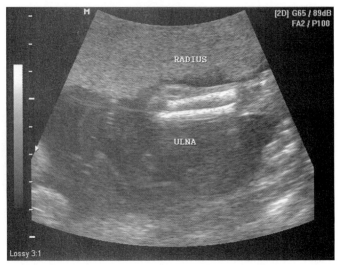

Fig. 17.13: Radius and ulna to be measured whenever a skeletal deformity is being suspected

- Hands (Fig. 17.14).

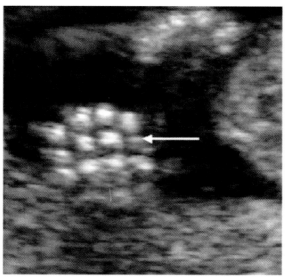

Fig. 17.14: The fifth digit should be carefully assessed for any incurving or any hypoplasia of the middle phalanx of the fifth digit (solid arrow)

SPECIFIC SKELETAL PARAMETERS FOR ASSESSING SKELETAL ABNORMALITIES

- Are the extremity bones abnormally short
  - Skeletal dysplasia
- Portions of bones are absent
  - Amputation
  - Radial ray defect
  - Sirenomelia.
- Extremities immobile or anomalously postured
  - Contractures
- Abnormalities of digits (hand or foot)
  - Polydactyly
  - Syndactyly.

Chapter 18

Anomalies of the Fetal Skeletal System

THANATOPHORIC DYSPLASIA

- The extremities are markedly short with the impression that the fetus is holding the extremities at right angles with the trunk (Fig. 18.1).
- Cloverleaf skull deformity with/without hydrocephalus.
- Bowed limbs giving a telephone receiver appearance.
- Cutaneous hydrops.
- Narrow thorax with extremely short ribs.
- Flattened vertebral bodies with wide disk spaces.

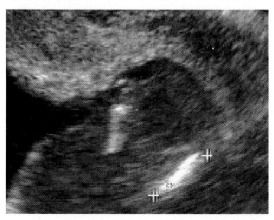

Fig. 18.1: Markedly short femur in a case of thanatophoric dysplasia. Bone lengths were corresponding to a size of 14 weeks in a fetus of 20 weeks gestation

ACHONDROGENESIS

- Severely retarded or absent skeletal ossification.
- Limb length reduction is quite severe.
- Short trunk and narrow thorax are present (Fig. 18.2).
- The lucent spinal column is unusually clear in the longitudinal section for the fetal spine.
- Depending on the severity of micromelia and the degree of vertebral body and calvarial ossification it is classified into two subtypes.

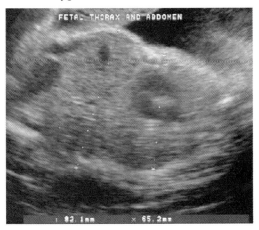

Fig. 18.2: Narrow thorax in a case of achondrogenesis. In the longitudinal section the anteroposterior diameter of the thorax is 65 mm and the anteroposterior diameter of the abdomen is 82 mm

OSTEOGENESIS IMPERFECTA

There are various types and subtypes but usual features seen on ultrasound are:

- Severe micromelia with crumpled irregular femurs (Fig. 18.3).
- Ribs are short and beaded secondary to fractures.
- Limb movement is limited.
- Fetal abdomen is protuberant.

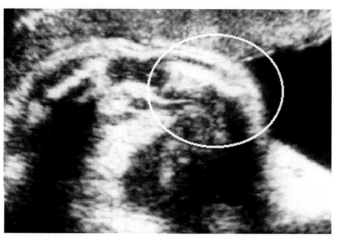

Fig. 18.3: Severe limb shortening with fractures (within circle) giving an appearance of crumpled long bones

ASPHYXIATING THORACIC DYSTROPHY

- Extremely narrow chest with secondary pulmonary hypoplasia (Fig. 18.4).
- Limbs could be mildly shortened or even of normal length.
- Polydactyly may be there.

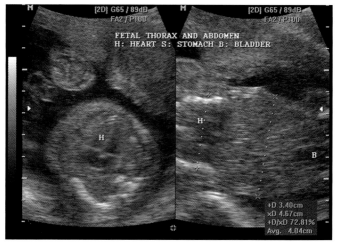

Fig. 18.4: Extremely narrow chest as seen in transverse and longitudinal measurements in a case of asphyxiating thorax dystrophy

CLUBFOOT (TALIPES)

- Can be unilateral or bilateral.
- The foot is usually turned medially.
- The best and simplest way to diagnose on ultrasound is to visualize the sole of the foot and if in this view one can see the tibia it is a clubfoot deformity (Fig. 18.5).
- Confirm the clubfoot deformity after the limb movement as the foot can sometimes be placed in such a manner giving the false impression of a club foot.

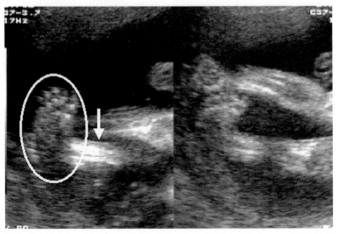

Fig. 18.5: Visualize the sole of the foot (within circle) and if in this view you can see the tibia (solid arrow); it is a clubfoot deformity

Chapter **19**

Fetal Hydrops

BASICS

All or any of the following:
- Pericardial effusion
- Pleural effusion
- Mediastinal effusion
- Ascites (Figs 19.2 and 19.3)
- Subcutaneous edema

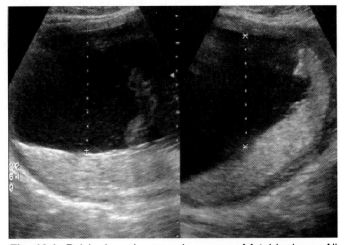

Fig. 19.1: Polyhydramnios seen in a case of fetal hydrops. All four quadrants (deepest vertical measurement) of the uterus are added up for assessing the liquor amnii and the amniotic fluid index is calculated. The AFI in this case was 292 mm

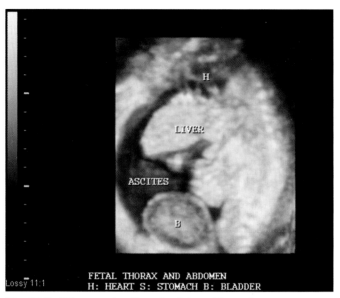

Fig. 19.2: 3D reconstruction of a fetus with ascites

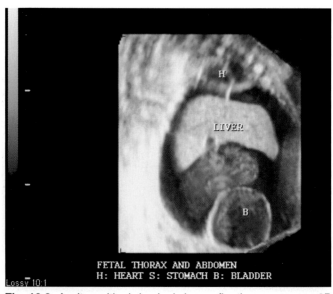

Fig. 19.3: Ascites with abdominal viscera floating as seen on 3D

• Hepatomegaly (Fig. 19.4)

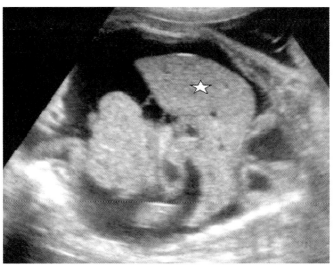

Fig. 19.4: Hepatomegaly (star), fetal liver is seen surrounded by ascitic fluid with associated pleural effusion and pericardial effusion

- Splenomegaly
- Placentomegaly
- Dilatation of the umbilical vein (Fig. 19.5)

These features are common to both immune and non-immune fetal hydrops.

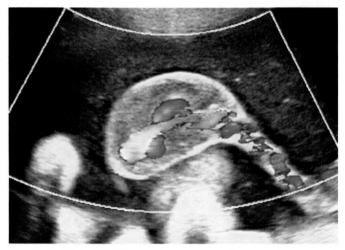

Fig. 19.5: Dilated umbilical vein and polyhydramnios in a case of fetal hydrops

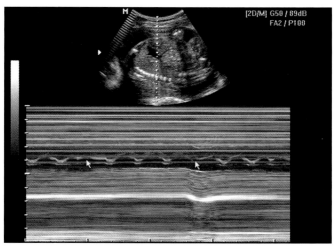

Fig. 19.6: Fetal M mode tracing showing missed beats in the cardiac rhythm. Note the pericardial effusion

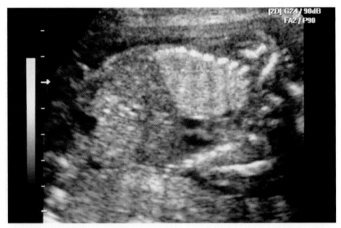

Fig. 19.7: Cystic adenomatoid malformation of the fetal lung

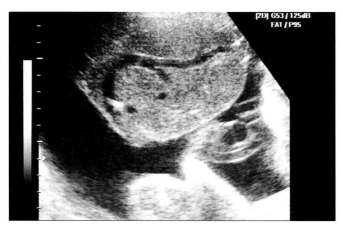

Fig. 19.8: Inhomogeneously hypoechoic large placental mass diagnosed as chorioangioma

BE CAREFULL OF

- Pseudoascites. Not infrequently in a transverse section the abdominal wall musculature can appear hypoechoic, mimicking ascites (Fig. 19.9).
- Differentiate cutaneous edema of a macrosomic fetus in a diabetic mother by checking for fetal biometry.
- Isolated nuchal skin fold thickening should not be diagnosed as fetal hydrops.
- Minimal normal pericardial fluid can often be seen.

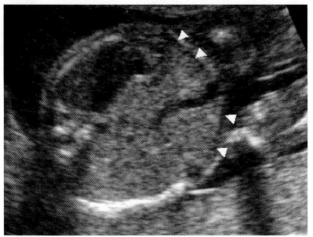

Fig. 19.9: Pseudoascites commonly seen in a transverse section is mostly seen anteriorly and does not outline the abdominal vasculature or viscera

Diagnosis of Fetal Malformations by Ultrasound in the First and Early Second Trimester

EMBRYOLOGIC DEVELOPMENT
AS SEEN ON ULTRASOUND

Advantages of transvaginal sonography over trans-abdominal route:
- Better resolution and visualization of early fetal/embryonic anatomy.
- Full bladder discomfort not required.
- Necessary in obese patients.
- Necessary in pregnancy in a retroverted uterus.
- Increased accuracy of measurements.
- Earlier diagnosis of anomalies.
- Earlier termination leads to less maternal and fetal bonding.

Disadvantages of transvaginal sonography:
- Maybe difficult to visualize due to unusual angles of presentation.
- Difficulty in apprehensive patient who may not allow proper transvaginal scanning.

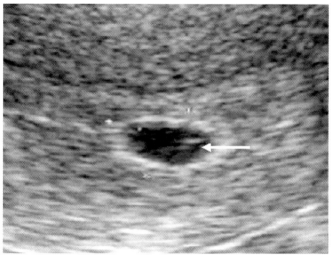

Fig. 20.1: Gestational sac of 5 weeks and 2 days with a yolk sac clearly delineated (solid arrow)

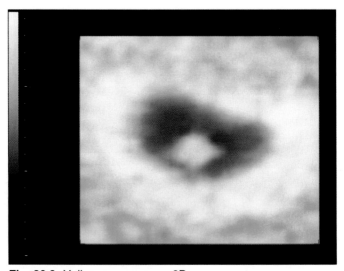

Fig. 20.2: Yolk sac as seen on 3D

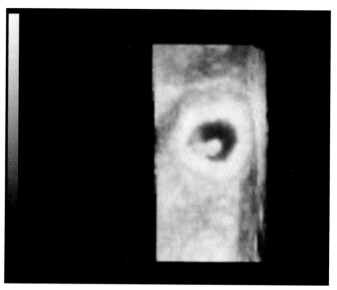

Fig. 20.3: 3D reconstruction of the gestational sac

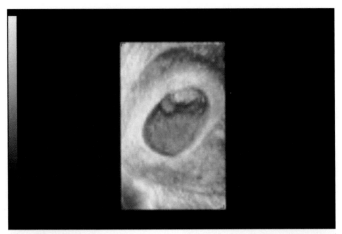

Fig. 20.4: 3D reconstruction of a 7 weeks 5 days embryo and yolk sac

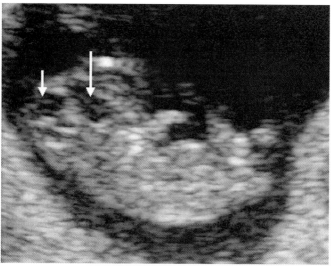

Fig. 20.5: Anechoic areas (solid arrows) seen in the brain of a fetus of 8 weeks and 6 days

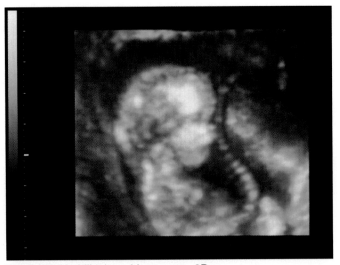

Fig. 20.6: Umbilical cord is seen on 3D

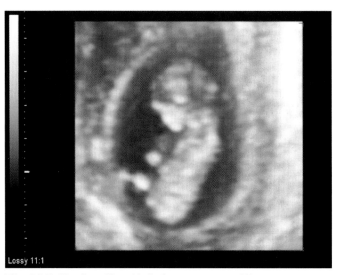

Lossy 11:1

Fig. 20.7: Fetal profile with limbs as seen on 3D

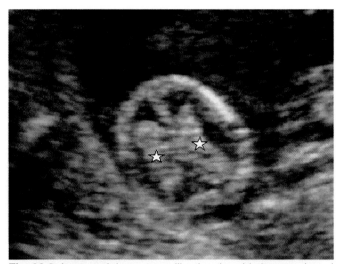

Fig. 20.8: Intracranial structures like the choroid plexuses (stars) delineated clearly for any early hydrocephalus or cysts

NUCHAL TRANSLUCENCY

Ultrasound appearances of an early pregnancy failure:
- > 5 mm embryo without cardiac activity
- > 8 mm gestational sac without a yolk sac
- >16 mm gestational sac without an embryo
- Flaccid, large or irregular amniotic sac.

Ultrasound appearances of an impending early pregnancy failure:
- Embryonic bradycardia in relation with the gestational age
- Oligoamniotic sac
- Interval sac growth poor
- Abnormal shape or size of yolk sac (Fig. 20.9).

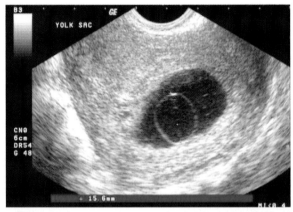

Fig. 20.9: Large yolk sec (15.6 mm) seen in the gestational sec

Embryonic time table and its appearances on ultrasound

Structures visible on ultrasound	No. of weeks from last menstrual period
Gestational sac	4w4d-5w0d
Yolk sac	5w0d-5w3d
Embryonic pole	5w2d
Cardiac pulsations	5w3d
Limb buds	8w0d and >
Fetal movements	8w0d and >
Bowel herniation	9w0d-11w0d
Kidneys	10w0d and >
Choroid plexus	10w0d and >
Calcification of calvarium	10w0d and >
Orbits	10w4d and >
Stomach bubble	11w0d and >
Cardiac configuration	12w0d and >
Urinary bladder	12w0d and >

Chapter 21

Fetal Anomalies in Chromosomal Aberrations

Fetal abnormalities in trisomy 21, 18 and 13

Organ system	Trisomy 21	Trisomy 18	Trisomy 13
Head and brain	Mild ventriculomegaly	Dolicocephaly Strawberry-shaped skull Large cisterna magna Choroid plexus cysts Agenesis of corpus callosum	Holoprosencephaly Agenesis of corpus callosum Ventriculomegaly Enlarged cisterna magna Microcephaly
Facial	Flat face Nasal bone Absent/Hypoplastic	Micrognathia Microphthalmia	Micrognathia Sloping forehead Cleft lip and/or palate Microphthalmia Hypotelorism
Neck	Thickened nuchal skin fold Cystic hygroma	Nuchal thickening	Nuchal thickening
Cardiac	Ventricular septal defect Atrial septal defects Atrioventricular canal Echogenic cardiac focus		Ventricular septal defect Atrial septal defect Dextrocardia Echogenic cardiac focus
Gastrointestinal	Hyperechoic bowel Esophageal atresia Duodenal atresia Diaphragmatic hernia	Diaphragmatic hernia Omphalocele Esophageal atresia	Omphalocele
Urogenital	Renal pyelectasis	Hydronephrosis,	Renal cortical cysts

Contd...

Contd...

Organ system	Trisomy 21	Trisomy 18	Trisomy 13
		Horseshoe kidney	Hydronephrosis Horseshoe kidney
Skeletal	Short femur and humerus Clinodactyly of fifth digit Widely spaced first and second toes Wide iliac angle	Clubfoot deformity Generalized arthrogryposis Clenched hands	Postaxial polydactyly Camptodactyly Overlapping digits
Hydrops/ cutaneous	Nonimmune hydrops		
Liquor amnii		Third trimester polyhydramnios	Third trimester hydramnios
Biometry		Second trimester—onset intrauterine growth retardation	Second trimester—onset intrauterine growth retardation
Doppler	Abnormal ductus venosus waveform	Abnormal ductus venosus waveform	Abnormal ductus venosus waveform
Figures	(Figs 21.1 to 21.13)	(Figs 21.5 to 21.7 and 21.12)	(Figs 21.5 to 21.7)

Fetal abnormalities in triploidy and Turner's syndrome

Organ system	Triploidy	XO
Head and brain	Ventriculomegaly Agenesis of the corpus callosum Dandy-Walker malformation Holoprosencephaly	
Spine	Meningomyelocele	
Facial	Hypertelorism Microphthalmia Micrognathia	
Neck	Cystic hygroma	Large, septate, cystic hygroma
Thorax		Pleural effusions
Cardiac	Septal defects	Coarctation of the aorta
Gastrointestinal	Omphalocele	Ascites
Urogenital	Hydronephrosis	Horseshoe kidneys
Skeletal	Syndactyly of the third and fourth fingers Clubbed feet	Short femur
Hydrops		Severe lymphedema of all the soft tissues
Placenta	Enlarged placenta or small, prematurely calcified placenta	
Liquor amnii	Oligohydramnios	
Biometry	Severe, early-onset, asymmetric intrauterine growth restriction(affecting the skeleton more than the head)	
Doppler	Abnormal umbilical artery Doppler waveform, showing a high-resistance pattern	

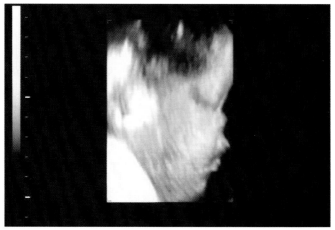

Fig. 21.1: Flat face with depressed nose as seen on 3D

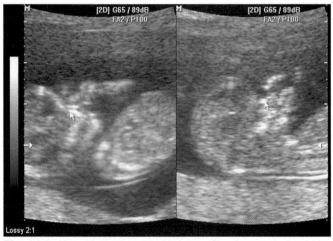

Fig. 21.2: Nasal bone is seen in the profile view and should be present in the scan done at 11-14 weeks

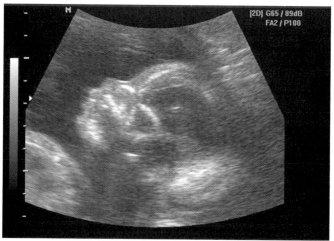

Fig. 21.3: An = (equal to) sign is made with the nasal bone and skin anterior to it

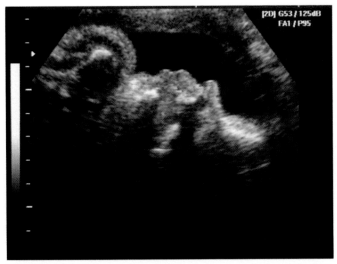

Fig. 21.4: Nasal bone absent in the late second trimester scan

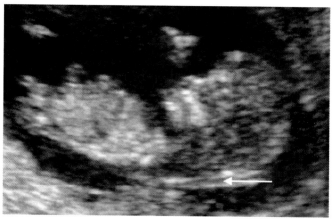

Fig. 21.5: Nuchal translucency: The *translucency* (subcutaneous) (solid arrow) between the skin and soft tissue posterior to the cervical spine has to be measured. Nuchal translucency thickness usually increases with gestational age with 1.5 mm and 2.5 mm being the 50th and 95th percentile respectively for gestational ages between 10 and 12 weeks. 2.0 mm and 3.0 mm are the 50th and 95th percentile respectively for gestational ages between 12 and 14 weeks

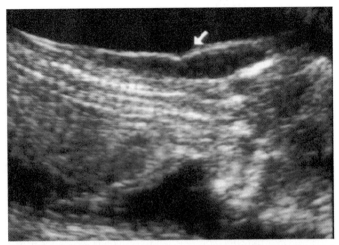

Fig. 21.6: A thickened nuchal translucency with spontaneous resolution and a normal nuchal skin fold thickness does not exclude a karyotypic abnormality. High-risk patients for chromosomal abnormalities and cardiac defects should definitely be subjected to an ultrasound between 10 and 14 weeks for measurement of nuchal translucency thickness

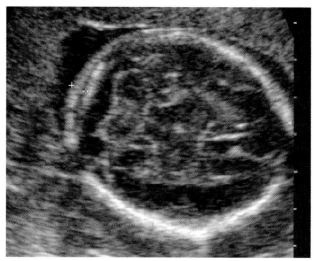

Fig. 21.7: The nuchal skin fold is measured from the posterior edge of the occipital bone and it includes the skin and the sonolucent area between the occipital bone and skin. Look in for any focal or diffuse thickening with/without septations

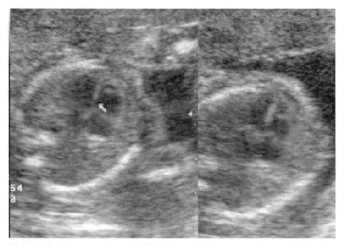

Fig. 21.8: Ventricular septal defect (arrow) seen in a trisomy 21 fetus with an associated thickened nuchal skin fold and short bone lengths

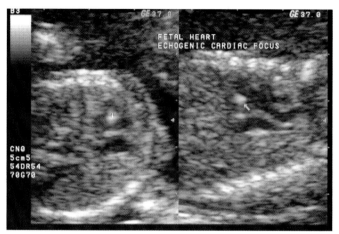

Fig. 21.9: Echogenic intracardiac focus seen in the fetal left ventricle

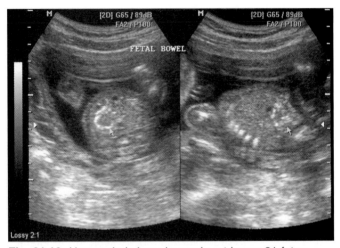

Fig. 21.10: Hyperechoic bowel seen in a trisomy 21 fetus

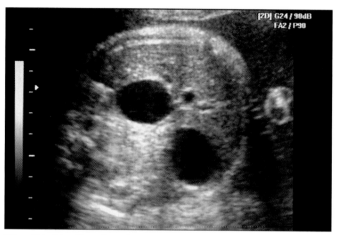

Fig. 21.11: Duodenal atresia (double bubble) seen in a trisomy 21 fetus

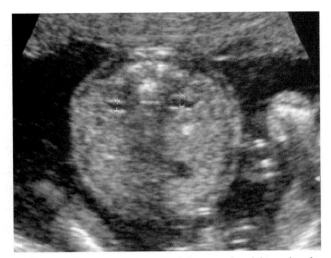

Fig. 21.12: The measurement of the renal pelvis varies from gestational age. The values for the anteroposterior diameter of the renal pelvis (a transverse view through the kidney). From 15-20 weeks of gestation < 04 mm is normal, 04-07 mm is borderline and > 08 mm is abnormal or hydronephrotic. From 20 weeks onwards < 06 mm is normal, 06-09 is borderline and > 10 mm is abnormal or hydronephrotic. Borderline cases are to be reviewed by serial scans before labelling them as hydronephrotic. Associated caliectasis or ureteric dilatation and whether unilateral or bilateral should definitely be looked for

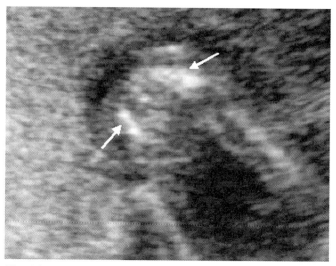

Fig. 21.13: Iliac bones (solid arrows) are normally seen at an angle of 60-75 degrees. 75-90 degrees is borderline and more than 90 degrees is a soft marker for trisomy 21

Chapter 22

Fetal Anomalies in Maternal Infections

Fetal abnormalities in maternal infections

Organ system	Cytomegalovirus	Rubella	Toxoplasmosis	Parvovirus
Head and brain	Ventriculomegaly Intracranial calcifications Microcephaly	Microcephaly	Ventriculomegaly Microcephaly Intracranial calcifications	
Facial		Cataracts Microphthalmia	Cataracts	
Cardiac	Cardiomegaly	Septal defects		Pericardial effusion
Gastrointestinal	Hyperechoic bowel Ascites Intrahepatic calcifications Hydrops	Enlarged liver and spleen	Intrahepatic calcifications Hepatomegaly Ascites	Ascites
Hydrops Placenta			Thickened placenta	Hydrops Thickened placenta
Liquor amnii Biometry	Intrauterine growth restriction	Intrauterine growth restriction	Intrauterine growth restriction	Polyhydramnios
Figures	(Figs 22.1 and 22.2)		(Figs 22.1 to 22.3)	(Figs 22.3 and 22.4)

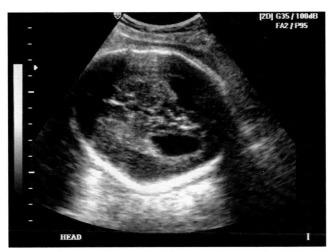

Fig. 22.1: Ventriculomegaly which can be seen in CMV and toxoplasmosis infection

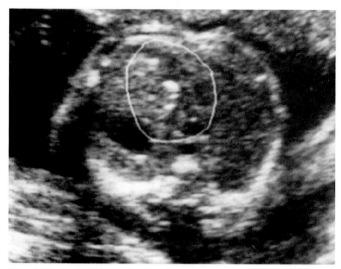

Fig. 22.2: Intrahepatic calcifications can be seen in cytomegalovirus and toxoplasmosis infection

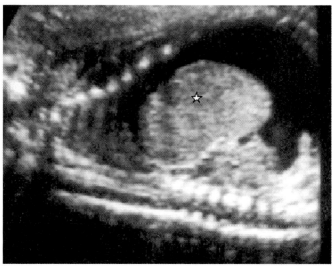

Fig. 22.3: Hepatomegaly (star) and ascites can be seen in rubella, toxoplasmosis and parvovirus infection

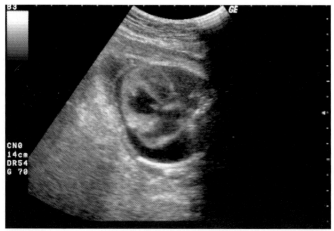

Fig. 22.4: Pericardial effusion which can be seen in parvovirus infection

Appendices

APPENDIX 1
Normal Values

NUCHAL TRANSLUCENCY

- Nuchal translucency thickness usually increases with gestational age.
- 1.5 mm and 2.5 mm are the 50th and 95th percentile respectively for gestational ages between 10 and 12 weeks.
- 2.0 mm and 3.0 mm are the 50th and 95th percentile respectively for gestational ages between 12 and 14 weeks.

NUCHAL SKIN FOLD

- (*14-18 weeks:* Normal value < 04 mm, borderline 04-05 mm and > 05 mm requires further karyotypic analysis).
- (*18-22 weeks:* Normal value < 05 mm, borderline 05-06 mm and > 06 mm requires further karyotypic analysis).
- After 22 weeks the sensitivity of nuchal skin fold thickness measurement for predicting karyotypic abnormalities is poor.

RENAL PELVIS

- The values for the anteroposterior diameter of the renal pelvis (measured on a transverse view through the kidney).

- From 15-20 weeks of gestation < 04 mm is normal, 04-07 mm is borderline and > 08 mm is abnormal or hydronephrotic.
- From 20 weeks onwards < 06 mm is normal, 06-09 is borderline and > 10 mm is abnormal or hydronephrotic.
- Borderline cases are to be reviewed by serial scans before labelling them as hydronephrotic. Check for caliectasis or ureteric dilatation.

VENTRICULAR ATRIUM

- The width of the body, anterior horn and posterior horn of the lateral ventricle are taken.
- (Normal value < 08 mm, borderline 08-10 mm and > 10 mm abnormal).
- When the choroid plexus does not occupy the whole of the body of the lateral ventricle see for the measurement of the medial separation of the choroid plexus from the wall of the lateral ventricle.
- (Normal value < 02 mm, borderline 02-03 mm and > 03 mm is abnormal).

CEREBELLAR TRANSVERSE DIAMETER

The CTD in mm from 14-22 weeks is equal to the gestational age of the fetus in weeks.

CISTERNA MAGNA

(Normal value < 08 mm, borderline 08-10 mm and > 10 mm abnormal).

SMALL BOWEL

Small bowel segments usually are less than 07 mm in diameter.

LARGE BOWEL

A large bowel segment which is more than 20 mm wide near term can be termed as abnormal.

PERICARDIAL FLUID

Minimal pericardial fluid is a normal finding after 20 weeks of gestation. So pericardial fluid of more than 02 mm is regarded as abnormal.

CUTANEOUS THICKNESS

Subcutaneous edema is diagnosed as abnormal when it measures more than 05 mm.

APPENDIX 2
Measurement Methodology

AMNIOTIC FLUID INDEX ASSESSMENT

The uterus is divided into four quadrants by the midline and transverse axis and the amniotic fluid as the deepest vertical pocket free of fetal parts and umbilical cord is measured in each quadrant and all four quadrants add up to give the amniotic fluid index.

CHOROID PLEXUS

Choroid plexus occupies the whole of the body of the lateral ventricle. The anterior horn, body and posterior horn of the lateral ventricle should be measured. Measurement of any medial separation of the choroids plexus with the lateral ventricular wall should also be assessed for.

CEREBELLUM

The cerebellum is seen as a 'W' turned 90 degrees. The cerebellar hemispheres and the cerebellar vermis should be appreciated for posterior cranial fossa abnormalities. The cerebellar transverse diameter (CTD) is measured from the edges of both cerebellar hemispheres.

CISTERNA MAGNA

The cisterna magna is seen posterior to the cerebellar vermis and anterior to the occipital bone.

NUCHAL TRANSLUCENCY

The translucency (subcutaneous) between the skin and soft tissue posterior to the cervical spine has to be measured.

NUCHAL SKIN

The nuchal skin fold is measured from the posterior edge of the occipital bone and it includes the skin and the sonolucent area between the occipital bone and skin. Look in for any focal or diffuse thickening with/without septations.

CRANIAL BIOMETRY

Section for cranial biometry consists of the thalamus, the third ventricle and the cavum septum pellucidum.

- *Biparietal diameter:* Side-to-side measurement from the outer table of the proximal skull to the inner table of the distal skull.
- *Head perimeter:* The total cranial circumference, which includes the maximum anteroposterior diameter.

- *Occipitofrontal diameter:* Front to back measurement from the outer table on both sides.

ORBITAL MEASUREMENTS

- *Ocular diameter:* Measured from medial inner to medial lateral wall of the long orbit.
- *Interocular distance:* Measured from medial inner wall of one orbit to medial inner wall of the other orbit.
- *Binocular distance:* Measured from lateral inner wall of one orbit to lateral inner wall of the other orbit.

ABDOMINAL PERIMETER

In the section for abdominal perimeter measurement,the spine should be posterior and the umbilical part of the portal vein anterior.

APPENDIX 3
Reporting

These are the parameters to be mentioned in the report. The list might appear too long but it is simple and one should routinely evaluate all these parameters.

Parameters to be routinely evaluated are mentioned as (R) and ones to be specifically looked in particular conditions are mentioned as (S).

FROM 05-10 WEEKS

- Uterine size (R)
- Location of gestational sac (R)
- Number of gestational sacs (R)
- Size of gestational sac (R)
- Yolk sac (R)
- Size of yolk sac (R)
- Embryo/fetus size (R)
- Menstrual age (R)
- Cardiac activity (R)
- Heart rate (R)
- Fetal movements (R)
- Trophoblastic reaction (R)
- Internal os width (R)
- Length of cervix (R)

- Any uterine mass (R)
- Any adnexal mass (R)
- Corpus luteum (present/absent) (R)
- Corpus luteum vascularity (S).

FROM 10-14 WEEKS

- Placental site (R)
- Liquor amnii (R)
- Fetal crown rump length (R)
- Menstrual age (R)
- Fetal movements and cardiac activity (R)
- Any gross anomalies (R)
- Nuchal translucency (R)
- Nasal bone (S)
- Ductus venosus flow (S)
- Internal os width (R)
- Length of cervix (R)
- Any uterine mass (R)
- Any adnexal mass (R).

FROM 14-22 WEEKS

- Placenta (R)
- Liquor amnii (R)
- Umbilical cord (R)
- Cervix (R)
- Lower segment (R)

- Myometrium (R)
- Adnexa (R)
- Nuchal skin thickness (S)
- Nasal bone (S)
- Cerebellar transverse diameter (S)
- Cisterna magna depth (S)
- Width of body of lateral ventricle (S)
- Inter-hemispheric distance (S)
- Ratio of the width of body of lateral ventricle to inter-hemispheric distance (S)
- Ocular diameter (S)
- Interocular distance (S)
- Binocular distance (S)
- Biparietal diameter (R)
- Occipitofrontal distance (R)
- Head perimeter (R)
- Abdominal perimeter (R)
- Femoral length (R)
- Humeral length (S)
- Foot length (S)
- Fetal movements and cardiac activity (R)
- Ductus venosus flow velocity waveform (S).

FROM 22-28 WEEKS

- All parameters of 14-22 weeks except nuchal skin fold thickness (R) and (S)

- Umbilical artery and uterine artery flow velocity waveform (S).

FROM 28-41 WEEKS

- Placenta (R)
- Liquor amnii (R)
- Umbilical cord (R)
- Cervix (R)
- Lower segment (R)
- Myometrium (R)
- Adnexa (R)
- Biparietal diameter (R)
- Occipitofrontal distance (R)
- Head perimeter (R)
- Abdominal perimeter (R)
- Femoral length (R)
- Distal femoral epiphysis (R)
- Biophysical profile (S)
- Color Doppler arterial (Umbilical artery, middle cerebral artery, descending aorta and both maternal uterine arteries) (S)
- Color Doppler venous (Umbilical vein, inferior vena cava and ductus venosus) (S).

Index

Fetal Anomalies

D

Dandy-Walker malformation 28
Diastematomyelia 85
Duodenal atresia 123

E

Echogenic bowel 126
Embryologic development as
    seen on ultrasound 176
Encephalocele 16
Esophageal atresia 122
Exencephaly (acrania) 12

F

Fetal abdomen (approach) 116
Fetal anomalies in maternal
    infections 207

G

Gastroschisis 128

H

Hydranencephaly 30
Hydronephrosis 137
Hypotelorism 55

I

Iniencephaly 20

K

Kidneys 132

L

Large bowel 216
Large bowel obstruction 127
Lips 44
Lobar 24
Longitudinal planes 73
Lung sequestration 96

M

Mandible 44
Maxilla 44
Micrognathia 57
Microphthalmia 59
Multicystic dysplastic kidney 141

N

Nasal bone 44, 60
Normal heart 102
Nuchal skin 218
Nuchal skin fold 65, 214
Nuchal translucency 64, 185,
    214, 218

O

Omphalocele 129

Index